Disclaimer:

The information presented in this book is for educational purposes only and is not intended to diagnose, treat, cure or prevent any disease. The contents of this book are based on research and the author's personal experience with healthy eating, and are not intended as a substitute for professional medical advice, diagnosis or treatment.

Please consult your healthcare provider before making any changes to your diet, particularly if you have any pre-existing medical conditions or are taking medication. Any reliance you place on the information presented in this book is strictly at your own risk.

The author and publisher of this book are not responsible for any adverse effects or consequences resulting from the use of any of the information or suggestions provided in this book. The reader should use their own judgement and consult with their own healthcare provider before implementing any dietary changes or making any other health-related decisions.

Chapter 1: Introduction to Healthy Eating

Healthy eating is not just about counting calories or restricting yourself to a certain type of food. It is about nourishing your body with wholesome, nutrient-dense foods that provide you with energy, improve your overall health, and help prevent chronic diseases. Healthy eating can also help you maintain a healthy weight and improve your mental health and cognitive function.

At its core, healthy eating involves consuming a balanced diet that includes a variety of foods from all food groups. This includes fruits, vegetables, whole grains, lean proteins, healthy fats, and low-fat dairy products. It is important to note that not all foods are created equal, and some provide more nutritional value than others. For example, a whole-grain bread will provide more fiber and nutrients than a slice of white bread.

A healthy diet should also be low in saturated and trans fats, added sugars, and sodium. These ingredients can increase the risk of heart disease, high blood pressure, and obesity. It is important to limit the consumption of processed foods, as they are often high in these unhealthy ingredients.

In addition to the types of food you eat, it is also important to consider how you eat. Eating mindfully, taking time to savor your food and listen to your body's hunger and fullness signals, can help you better control your portions and avoid overeating. Drinking plenty of water throughout the day can also help you stay hydrated and prevent overeating.

Making healthy food choices can seem overwhelming, but it doesn't have to be. Small changes, such as swapping out soda for water or adding more vegetables to your meals, can have a big impact on your health over time. It is also important to remember that healthy eating is a lifestyle, not a temporary diet. It is about creating sustainable habits that you can stick to in the long term.

In this book, we will explore the different aspects of healthy eating, from macronutrients and micronutrients to the benefits of whole foods and plant-based diets. We will also discuss the dangers of processed foods and added sugars, and provide practical tips for incorporating healthy eating into your busy lifestyle. By the end of this book, you will have a better understanding of what it means to eat healthy, and be equipped with the knowledge and tools to make informed decisions about your diet.

Chapter 2: Benefits of a Healthy Diet

Eating a healthy diet is one of the most important things you can do for your overall health and well-being. A healthy diet is one that is rich in nutrients, low in processed foods and added sugars, and is balanced to meet your individual needs. Here are some of the many benefits of a healthy diet:

Weight management: Eating a healthy diet can help you maintain a healthy weight or even lose weight if you need to. A diet that is high in fruits, vegetables, whole grains, lean proteins, and healthy fats can help you feel full and satisfied, which can prevent overeating and weight gain.

Better digestion: A healthy diet that is rich in fiber can promote good digestive health. Fiber helps keep your digestive system regular, prevents constipation, and can even reduce your risk of developing certain digestive disorders.

Improved heart health: A diet that is high in fruits, vegetables, whole grains, and lean proteins can help reduce your risk of heart disease. These foods are low in saturated and trans fats, which can raise your cholesterol levels and increase your risk of heart disease.

Reduced risk of chronic diseases: Eating a healthy diet can help reduce your risk of chronic diseases, such as type 2 diabetes, certain types of cancer, and Alzheimer's disease. Foods that are high in antioxidants and anti-inflammatory compounds, such as fruits, vegetables, nuts, and seeds, can help protect your body from the damage that can lead to these diseases.

Improved mood: What you eat can also affect your mood and mental health. A diet that is high in nutrients, such as omega-3 fatty acids, B vitamins, and magnesium, can help improve your mood and reduce symptoms of depression and anxiety.

Increased energy: Eating a healthy diet can also help boost your energy levels. A diet that is rich in complex carbohydrates, such as whole grains, and protein can provide your body with the fuel it needs to stay energized throughout the day.

Better sleep: What you eat can also affect your sleep quality. A diet that is high in foods that contain tryptophan, such as turkey, chicken, bananas, and nuts, can help promote better sleep.

In conclusion, the benefits of a healthy diet are numerous and can have a significant impact on your overall health and well-being. By making small changes to your diet, such as incorporating more fruits, vegetables, and whole grains, you can improve your health and reduce your risk of chronic diseases.

Chapter 3: Macronutrients and Micronutrients

When it comes to eating healthy, understanding the difference between macronutrients and micronutrients is essential. Macronutrients are the nutrients that provide energy to your body, while micronutrients are essential for your body to function properly.

Macronutrients include carbohydrates, proteins, and fats. Carbohydrates are the primary source of energy for your body, and they are found in foods such as bread, pasta, rice, and fruits. Proteins are essential for building and repairing tissues in your body, and they are found in foods such as meat, fish, eggs, and beans. Fats are also a source of energy for your body, and they are found in foods such as nuts, seeds, avocados, and oils.

While macronutrients provide the energy that your body needs to function, micronutrients are essential for your body to carry out its everyday processes. Micronutrients include vitamins and minerals, and they are found in a variety of foods such as fruits, vegetables, dairy products, and meats.

Vitamins are organic compounds that your body needs in small amounts to carry out specific functions. For example, vitamin C is essential for the health of your immune system, while vitamin A is important for maintaining healthy vision. Minerals, on the other hand, are inorganic compounds that your body needs in small amounts to carry out specific functions. For example, calcium is essential for maintaining strong bones, while iron is important for the production of red blood cells.

Eating a balanced diet that includes a variety of foods from each food group can help ensure that you are getting all of the macronutrients and micronutrients that your body needs. It is important to note that different foods contain different amounts of macronutrients and micronutrients, so it is important to pay attention to what you are eating to ensure that you are getting a balanced diet.

In addition to eating a balanced diet, it may be helpful to take a multivitamin supplement to ensure that you are getting all of the micronutrients that your body needs. However, it is important to talk to your healthcare provider before taking any supplements to ensure that they are safe for you to take.

Overall, understanding the difference between macronutrients and micronutrients is essential for maintaining a healthy diet. By eating a balanced diet that includes a variety of foods from each food group, you can ensure that your body is getting all of the nutrients that it needs to function properly.

Chapter 4: The Importance of Water

Water is a vital component of our body and a crucial element in maintaining good health. It is essential for the proper functioning of our body and plays a crucial role in various bodily functions.

Water helps to regulate our body temperature, lubricate our joints, transport nutrients and oxygen to cells, and remove waste and toxins from our body. It is also crucial for the proper functioning of our digestive system and aids in the absorption of nutrients from the food we eat.

One of the most important reasons why water is essential for good health is that it helps to keep our bodies hydrated. Dehydration can lead to a host of health problems, including headaches, fatigue, constipation, and kidney stones. It can also affect our mood and cognitive function, making it difficult to concentrate and perform tasks.

Drinking enough water is especially important for people who engage in physical activity or live in hot climates. When we sweat, we lose water, and if we do not replace it, we can become dehydrated, which can be dangerous. Athletes and people who engage in strenuous exercise need to drink more water to replace the fluids lost during exercise.

Water is also an excellent alternative to sugary drinks, which can be high in calories and lead to weight gain. Drinking water can help to fill us up and reduce our appetite, making it easier to maintain a healthy weight. It is also important to note that water does not contain any calories or sugar, making it an ideal beverage for people who want to reduce their sugar intake.

Furthermore, water is an essential part of a healthy diet. Drinking water before meals can help to reduce our appetite and prevent overeating, which can contribute to weight gain. Water is also an excellent alternative to sugary beverages, which can increase the risk of obesity, type 2 diabetes, and other health problems.

In conclusion, water is an essential nutrient that is necessary for good health. It is essential for the proper functioning of our body and plays a crucial role in various bodily functions. Drinking enough water can help to keep us hydrated, maintain a healthy weight, and prevent a host of health problems. Therefore, it is important to make sure that we drink enough water every day to maintain good health.

Chapter 5: Fiber and Digestion

Fiber is an essential component of a healthy diet, and it plays a vital role in digestion. It is a type of carbohydrate that our body cannot digest, and therefore it passes through our digestive system relatively unchanged.

There are two types of fiber, soluble and insoluble. Soluble fiber dissolves in water, and it forms a gel-like substance in the digestive tract. It can be found in foods such as oats, beans, apples, and citrus fruits. Insoluble fiber does not dissolve in water, and it helps to add bulk to the stool. It can be found in foods such as whole grains, vegetables, and nuts.

Fiber plays a crucial role in digestion because it helps to regulate bowel movements and prevent constipation. When we eat fiber-rich foods, it adds bulk to the stool, making it easier to pass through the intestines. This can help to prevent constipation and other digestive issues such as hemorrhoids.

In addition to its role in preventing constipation, fiber also helps to regulate blood sugar levels. Soluble fiber, in particular, slows down the absorption of sugar in the bloodstream. This can help to prevent blood sugar spikes and dips, which can be harmful to those with diabetes or insulin resistance.

Fiber also helps to lower cholesterol levels. Soluble fiber binds to cholesterol in the digestive tract and helps to remove it from the body. This can help to lower LDL (bad) cholesterol levels and reduce the risk of heart disease.

It is important to consume an adequate amount of fiber in your diet. The recommended daily intake of fiber for adults is 25 grams for women and 38 grams for men. However, many people fall short of this goal. To increase your fiber intake, try incorporating more whole grains, fruits, vegetables, and legumes into your diet.

It is also important to increase your fiber intake gradually, as consuming too much fiber too quickly can cause digestive discomfort such as bloating and gas. It is recommended to increase your fiber intake slowly over a few weeks while also increasing your water intake to help prevent any digestive discomfort.

In conclusion, fiber plays an essential role in digestion and overall health. By consuming an adequate amount of fiber in your diet, you can help to regulate bowel movements, prevent constipation, regulate blood sugar levels, lower cholesterol levels, and reduce the risk of heart disease.

Chapter 6: The Truth about Carbohydrates

Carbohydrates are one of the three macronutrients that our body needs to function properly, alongside protein and fat. They are essential for providing energy to our body and brain, and they can be found in many different types of food such as fruits, vegetables, grains, and dairy products.

However, carbohydrates have also been the subject of much controversy in recent years, with some people claiming that they are the cause of weight gain, diabetes, and other health problems. In this chapter, we will explore the truth about carbohydrates and how they can fit into a healthy diet.

First, it is important to understand that not all carbohydrates are created equal. Carbohydrates can be divided into two categories: simple and complex. Simple carbohydrates are found in foods like candy, soda, and other sugary treats. They are made up of one or two sugar molecules and are quickly digested by the body, leading to a rapid increase in blood sugar levels. Complex carbohydrates, on the other hand, are found in foods like whole grains, beans, and vegetables. They are made up of long chains of sugar molecules and are digested more slowly, leading to a more gradual increase in blood sugar levels.

The type of carbohydrate you choose can have a big impact on your health. Foods high in simple carbohydrates, such as candy and soda, provide little nutritional value and can contribute to weight gain and other health problems. On the other hand, foods high in complex carbohydrates, such as whole grains, fruits, and vegetables, provide important nutrients like fiber, vitamins, and minerals, and can help maintain a healthy weight and prevent chronic diseases like diabetes and heart disease.

Another important factor to consider when it comes to carbohydrates is portion size. While complex carbohydrates can be a healthy part of a balanced diet, consuming too many carbohydrates can still lead to weight gain. This is because excess carbohydrates are converted into fat and stored in the body. It is important to choose appropriate portion sizes and balance carbohydrates with protein and healthy fats.

Finally, it is worth noting that some people may have specific dietary needs when it comes to carbohydrates. For example, people with diabetes may need to monitor their carbohydrate intake to manage their blood sugar levels. Additionally, some people may have difficulty digesting certain types of carbohydrates, such as those found in beans or wheat, and may need to avoid or limit these foods.

In conclusion, carbohydrates are an important part of a healthy diet, but it is important to choose the right types and consume them in appropriate portions. Simple carbohydrates found in sugary treats provide little nutritional value and can contribute to health problems, while complex carbohydrates found in whole grains, fruits, and vegetables can provide important nutrients and help maintain a healthy weight. By making smart choices about the types and portions of carbohydrates we consume, we can enjoy the many benefits of this essential nutrient while maintaining good health.

Chapter 7: Good Fats vs Bad Fats

When it comes to healthy eating, one of the most important considerations is the type of fats that you consume. Not all fats are created equal, and some can have a negative impact on your health, while others can actually be beneficial. In this chapter, we'll explore the differences between good fats and bad fats and provide you with the information you need to make informed choices about your diet.

What are Fats?

Fats are an essential part of a healthy diet. They provide energy, support cell growth, protect organs, and help to keep the body warm. There are three types of dietary fats: saturated, unsaturated, and trans fats. Saturated fats are typically solid at room temperature and are found in animal products such as meat, dairy, and butter. Unsaturated fats are liquid at room temperature and are typically found in plant-based foods such as nuts, seeds, and oils. Trans fats are found in processed foods such as baked goods, fried foods, and snack foods.

Good Fats

Good fats, also known as healthy fats, include monounsaturated and polyunsaturated fats. These fats can help to lower bad cholesterol levels, reduce inflammation, and improve heart health.

Monounsaturated fats can be found in foods such as avocados, nuts, and olive oil. They have been shown to help reduce the risk of heart disease by lowering bad cholesterol levels and increasing good cholesterol levels.

Polyunsaturated fats are found in foods such as fatty fish, flaxseed, and walnuts. They contain essential fatty acids, including omega-3 and omega-6, which the body needs but cannot produce on its own. Omega-3 fatty acids have been shown to reduce inflammation, lower blood pressure, and decrease the risk of heart disease.

Bad Fats

Bad fats, also known as unhealthy fats, include saturated and trans fats. These fats can increase bad cholesterol levels, raise the risk of heart disease, and contribute to inflammation.

Saturated fats are typically found in animal products such as meat, cheese, and butter. They can also be found in some plant-based foods such as coconut oil and palm oil. Consuming too much saturated fat can increase bad cholesterol levels and increase the risk of heart disease.

Trans fats are found in processed foods such as baked goods, fried foods, and snack foods. They are created through a process called hydrogenation, which turns liquid vegetable oil into a solid form. Trans fats have been shown to increase bad cholesterol levels and decrease good cholesterol levels, which can lead to an increased risk of heart disease.

Conclusion

In summary, not all fats are created equal. Consuming healthy fats, such as monounsaturated and polyunsaturated fats, can have a positive impact on your health by reducing bad cholesterol levels, lowering inflammation, and improving heart health. On the other hand, consuming unhealthy fats, such as saturated and trans fats, can have negative effects on your health by increasing bad cholesterol levels, raising the risk of heart disease, and contributing to inflammation. When making food choices, it's important to pay attention to the types of fats in your diet and make choices that prioritize healthy fats over unhealthy ones.

Chapter 8: The Benefits of Protein

Protein is an essential macronutrient that is critical for the proper functioning of the human body. It is a fundamental building block for muscles, bones, skin, and hair, and it plays a vital role in numerous biological processes. Incorporating protein into your diet is essential for optimal health, and it provides numerous benefits for your body.

One of the main benefits of protein is its ability to help with weight loss. Protein is known to be more filling than other macronutrients, such as carbohydrates and fats, and it can help reduce hunger and cravings. This can lead to a decrease in overall calorie intake, which can help you lose weight. Additionally, protein has a higher thermic effect than other macronutrients, which means that your body burns more calories digesting and processing it. This can also contribute to weight loss.

Protein is also essential for building and maintaining muscle mass. When you exercise, your muscles undergo stress and damage, and protein is required to repair and rebuild them. Adequate protein intake can help ensure that your body has the necessary building blocks to repair and grow muscle tissue. This is especially important for individuals who engage in strength training or other forms of high-intensity exercise.

In addition to its muscle-building properties, protein also plays a critical role in bone health. Bones are made up of a matrix of proteins and minerals, and adequate protein intake is necessary for maintaining strong, healthy bones. Studies have shown that individuals who consume higher amounts of protein have greater bone density and a lower risk of osteoporosis.

Protein is also important for maintaining healthy skin, hair, and nails. These structures are primarily made up of protein, and consuming adequate amounts of protein can help keep them strong and healthy. Additionally, protein is involved in the production of collagen, a protein that provides structure and elasticity to the skin.

Finally, protein is essential for numerous biological processes in the body, including the synthesis of hormones and enzymes. Hormones are responsible for regulating various bodily functions, such as metabolism, growth, and reproduction, and adequate protein intake is necessary for their production. Enzymes are essential for numerous chemical reactions in the body, and many of these enzymes are made up of protein.

In conclusion, protein is an essential macronutrient that provides numerous benefits for the human body. It is important for weight loss, muscle building, bone health, skin, hair, and nail health, and the synthesis of hormones and enzymes. Incorporating protein-rich foods into your diet, such as lean meats, fish, eggs, dairy products, legumes, and nuts, is essential for optimal health.

Chapter 9: Vitamins and Minerals

Vitamins and minerals are essential nutrients that our bodies need in small amounts to function properly. They are found in a wide variety of healthy foods, including fruits, vegetables, whole grains, and lean proteins. In this chapter, we will explore the importance of vitamins and minerals in our diet and the foods that are rich sources of these vital nutrients.

Vitamins are organic compounds that our bodies need to carry out various functions, such as supporting our immune system, promoting healthy skin, and helping us maintain strong bones. There are 13 essential vitamins that our bodies need, including vitamins A, C, D, E, K, and the B vitamins. Each vitamin plays a unique role in maintaining our overall health, and a deficiency in any one of these vitamins can lead to serious health problems.

Minerals, on the other hand, are inorganic substances that our bodies need for a variety of functions, including building strong bones, regulating our metabolism, and maintaining proper fluid balance. Some of the essential minerals that our bodies need include calcium, iron, magnesium, potassium, and zinc.

To ensure that we are getting enough vitamins and minerals in our diet, it is important to eat a variety of nutrient-rich foods. Fruits and vegetables are particularly good sources of vitamins and minerals, as they contain a wide range of nutrients that our bodies need to function properly.

For example, leafy green vegetables like spinach and kale are excellent sources of vitamins A, C, and K, as well as minerals like calcium and magnesium. Fruits like oranges and strawberries are rich in vitamin C, while berries and other colorful fruits are great sources of antioxidants, which help to protect our bodies from damage caused by harmful free radicals.

In addition to fruits and vegetables, whole grains are also important sources of vitamins and minerals. Whole grains like brown rice, quinoa, and oats are rich in B vitamins, iron, and magnesium, which are important for maintaining healthy energy levels and supporting our nervous system.

Lean proteins like chicken, fish, and legumes are also important sources of vitamins and minerals. For example, fish like salmon and tuna are rich in vitamin D and omega-3 fatty acids, which help to support our cardiovascular health and cognitive function. Legumes like lentils and chickpeas are good sources of iron, potassium, and magnesium, which are important for maintaining healthy muscles and bones.

In conclusion, vitamins and minerals are essential nutrients that our bodies need to function properly. By eating a varied diet that includes plenty of fruits, vegetables, whole grains, and lean proteins, we can ensure that we are getting enough of these vital nutrients to support our overall health and wellbeing.

Chapter 10: Phytonutrients and Antioxidants

Phytonutrients and antioxidants are two essential components found in healthy foods that offer numerous health benefits to the body. These nutrients are naturally occurring compounds that are present in plants and play a crucial role in the plant's growth and survival. When consumed by humans, they provide numerous health benefits, such as reducing the risk of chronic diseases, improving immune function, and promoting healthy aging.

Phytonutrients, also known as phytochemicals, are biologically active compounds that give plants their vibrant colors, smells, and flavors. These nutrients are found in a variety of foods, including fruits, vegetables, whole grains, legumes, nuts, and seeds. Phytonutrients have numerous health benefits, such as reducing inflammation, improving heart health, and reducing the risk of cancer.

There are many different types of phytonutrients, including carotenoids, flavonoids, and polyphenols. Carotenoids are pigments that give fruits and vegetables their bright colors, such as beta-carotene found in carrots and lycopene found in tomatoes. Flavonoids are found in fruits, vegetables, and dark chocolate and have antioxidant and anti-inflammatory properties. Polyphenols are found in fruits, vegetables, and tea and have been shown to improve heart health and cognitive function.

Antioxidants are another essential component found in healthy foods that help protect the body from damage caused by free radicals. Free radicals are unstable molecules that can damage cells, and antioxidants neutralize these harmful molecules before they can cause damage. Antioxidants are found in many different types of foods, including fruits, vegetables, nuts, and seeds.

There are several different types of antioxidants, including vitamin C, vitamin E, and beta-carotene. Vitamin C is found in citrus fruits, berries, and leafy greens and helps support the immune system and protect against infections. Vitamin E is found in nuts, seeds, and leafy greens and helps protect against heart disease and cancer. Beta-carotene is found in orange and yellow fruits and vegetables and is converted into vitamin A in the body, which is essential for healthy vision and skin.

In conclusion, consuming foods rich in phytonutrients and antioxidants is essential for maintaining good health and preventing chronic diseases. These nutrients are found in a variety of foods, including fruits, vegetables, whole grains, legumes, nuts, and seeds. By including a wide variety of these foods in your diet, you can reap the many health benefits associated with these essential nutrients.

Chapter 11: The Role of Enzymes in Digestion

Digestion is a complex process that involves breaking down food into smaller molecules that can be absorbed and utilized by the body. This process is aided by various enzymes that are produced in different parts of the digestive system. Enzymes are specialized proteins that speed up chemical reactions in the body without being consumed in the process.

Enzymes are essential for digestion because they break down large food molecules into smaller molecules that can be absorbed by the body. These smaller molecules are then used to provide energy and nutrients to the body's cells. Without enzymes, the digestive process would be slow and inefficient, and the body would not be able to extract the necessary nutrients from the food we eat.

The digestive system produces a variety of enzymes that are involved in different stages of digestion. These enzymes are produced in various organs such as the mouth, stomach, pancreas, and small intestine. Each enzyme is designed to break down a specific type of molecule. For example, amylase is an enzyme produced in the mouth and pancreas that breaks down carbohydrates into smaller sugars, while lipase is an enzyme produced in the pancreas that breaks down fats into smaller fatty acids.

The digestive process begins in the mouth, where food is mechanically broken down by chewing and mixed with saliva. Saliva contains an enzyme called amylase, which begins to break down carbohydrates into smaller sugars. Once food is swallowed, it enters the stomach, where it is mixed with stomach acid and digestive enzymes. The stomach produces several enzymes, including pepsin, which breaks down proteins into smaller peptides.

After leaving the stomach, food enters the small intestine, where the majority of digestion and nutrient absorption takes place. The pancreas secretes digestive enzymes into the small intestine, including amylase, lipase, and protease. These enzymes help to break down carbohydrates, fats, and proteins into smaller molecules that can be absorbed by the body's cells.

Enzymes play a crucial role in digestion, but certain factors can affect their function. For example, a diet that is high in processed foods and low in fiber can lead to a reduction in digestive enzymes, which can make it harder for the body to break down and absorb nutrients. In addition, certain medications, such as antibiotics, can disrupt the balance of gut bacteria, which can affect the production of digestive enzymes.

To promote healthy digestion, it is important to eat a diet that is rich in whole, nutrient-dense foods and to avoid processed and refined foods. This can help to ensure that the body has the necessary enzymes and nutrients to efficiently break down and absorb food. In addition, consuming fermented foods, such as yogurt and sauerkraut, can help to promote the growth of beneficial gut bacteria, which can enhance the production of digestive enzymes.

In conclusion, enzymes play a crucial role in the digestive process by breaking down food into smaller molecules that can be absorbed and utilized by the body. A diet that is rich in whole, nutrient-dense foods and that supports the growth of beneficial gut bacteria can help to ensure that the body has the necessary enzymes and nutrients to efficiently digest and absorb food.

Chapter 12: The Connection Between Diet and Disease

Diet and disease are closely interconnected. The food we eat plays a significant role in determining our overall health and well-being. Poor dietary choices can lead to a range of chronic diseases, including heart disease, diabetes, obesity, and certain types of cancer.

There are several factors that contribute to the connection between diet and disease. One of the most important factors is the nutritional content of the foods we eat. Nutrients like vitamins, minerals, and fiber are essential for maintaining optimal health. A diet that is rich in these nutrients can help reduce the risk of chronic diseases and improve overall health.

On the other hand, diets that are high in saturated fats, processed foods, and refined sugars can have a negative impact on health. These types of foods have been linked to an increased risk of heart disease, diabetes, and obesity. They can also contribute to inflammation in the body, which can lead to a range of chronic diseases.

Another factor that plays a role in the connection between diet and disease is the way that food is processed and prepared. For example, cooking methods that involve high heat, such as grilling or frying, can produce harmful compounds that increase the risk of cancer. Similarly, foods that are heavily processed or contain artificial additives can have negative health effects.

The timing and frequency of meals can also impact health. Skipping meals or eating irregularly can disrupt the body's natural rhythms and lead to hormonal imbalances, which can contribute to a range of health problems. On the other hand, eating regular, balanced meals can help maintain optimal health and reduce the risk of chronic disease.

Finally, it is worth noting that individual genetics and lifestyle factors can also play a role in the connection between diet and disease. For example, certain genetic variations may make some people more susceptible to certain types of chronic diseases, regardless of their dietary choices. Additionally, factors like stress, sleep, and physical activity can all impact overall health and disease risk.

In conclusion, the connection between diet and disease is complex and multifaceted. However, it is clear that the foods we eat play a significant role in determining our overall health and well-being. By making smart dietary choices and prioritizing nutrient-rich, whole foods, we can help reduce our risk of chronic diseases and improve our quality of life.

Chapter 13: Eating for Energy

We all know that feeling of sluggishness that creeps in after a heavy meal or a long day at work. Our bodies need energy to function properly, and the food we eat plays a critical role in providing that energy. Eating for energy is all about choosing the right foods that will fuel your body and keep you feeling alert and energized throughout the day.

Complex Carbohydrates

One of the best ways to get a sustained source of energy is by consuming complex carbohydrates. These are the types of carbohydrates that take longer to break down and provide a slow release of energy throughout the day. Complex carbohydrates include whole grains like brown rice, whole wheat bread, and quinoa, as well as starchy vegetables like sweet potatoes and squash. These foods are also rich in fiber, which helps regulate blood sugar levels and prevents energy crashes.

Lean Protein

Protein is essential for building and repairing tissues in the body, but it also plays a role in providing energy. When we eat protein, our bodies break it down into amino acids, which can be used to produce glucose, the primary source of fuel for our cells. Lean protein sources like chicken, fish, tofu, and legumes are excellent choices for sustained energy throughout the day.

Healthy Fats

Contrary to popular belief, not all fats are bad for you. In fact, healthy fats can provide a long-lasting source of energy and help you feel fuller for longer periods of time. Healthy fat sources include avocados, nuts, seeds, olive oil, and fatty fish like salmon. These fats are also important for brain function and can help improve cognitive function.

Hydration

Drinking enough water is crucial for maintaining energy levels. Even mild dehydration can cause fatigue and lethargy, so it's important to drink water throughout the day. In addition to water, you can also consume water-rich foods like fruits and vegetables, which can help you stay hydrated and energized.

Balanced Meals

Finally, eating balanced meals is essential for maintaining energy levels throughout the day. A balanced meal should include complex carbohydrates, lean protein, healthy fats, and plenty of fruits and vegetables. Avoiding processed foods and sugary snacks can also help prevent energy crashes and keep you feeling energized.

In conclusion, eating for energy is all about choosing the right foods that will provide sustained energy throughout the day. Complex carbohydrates, lean protein, healthy fats, hydration, and balanced meals are all key components of a healthy and energizing diet. By making these simple changes to your diet, you can improve your energy levels, feel more alert and productive, and enjoy a healthier, happier life.

Chapter 14: Eating for Mental Clarity

Eating the right foods can have a significant impact on your mental clarity and overall cognitive function. A healthy diet can help reduce brain fog, improve memory retention, enhance concentration, and promote a more positive mood. In this chapter, we will explore some of the best foods for promoting mental clarity and how you can incorporate them into your diet.

Omega-3 Fatty Acids

Omega-3 fatty acids are essential fats that cannot be produced by the body and must be obtained through diet.

They are important for brain function and help reduce inflammation, which can contribute to cognitive decline. Foods rich in omega-3s include fatty fish such as salmon, mackerel, and sardines, as well as chia seeds, flaxseeds, and walnuts. Aim to eat at least two servings of fatty fish per week, or consider taking an omega-3 supplement.

Berries

Berries are rich in antioxidants and other compounds that help protect the brain from oxidative stress. They also contain flavonoids, which can improve cognitive function and memory. Blueberries, in particular, have been shown to improve brain function and delay age-related cognitive decline. Other berries to consider include strawberries, raspberries, and blackberries.

Leafy Greens

Leafy greens such as kale, spinach, and collard greens are packed with vitamins and minerals that are essential for brain health. They are also rich in antioxidants and other compounds that help reduce inflammation and protect the brain from damage. Aim to include at least one serving of leafy greens in your diet each day, whether it be in a salad, smoothie, or stir-fry.

Nuts and Seeds

Nuts and seeds are a great source of healthy fats, protein, and fiber. They also contain vitamins and minerals that are important for brain health, such as vitamin E and magnesium. Almonds, cashews, and pumpkin seeds are all good options to consider. Just be sure to opt for unsalted varieties to keep your sodium intake in check.

Whole Grains

Whole grains such as brown rice, quinoa, and oats are a good source of complex carbohydrates that provide a steady source of energy to the brain. They also contain fiber, vitamins, and minerals that are important for brain health. Aim to include at least one serving of whole grains in your diet each day, whether it be in the form of a bowl of oatmeal, a quinoa salad, or a serving of brown rice.

In conclusion, eating a healthy diet that is rich in omega-3 fatty acids, berries, leafy greens, nuts and seeds, and whole grains can help promote mental clarity and overall cognitive function. By incorporating these foods into your diet on a regular basis, you can help reduce brain fog, improve memory retention, enhance concentration, and promote a more positive mood. So the next time you're at the grocery store, be sure to load up on these brain-boosting foods!

Chapter 15: Eating for Strong Bones

Strong bones are vital for a healthy body, and good

nutrition plays a crucial role in maintaining bone health. Bones are not static structures; they are continuously breaking down and rebuilding. In order to maintain strong bones, we need to provide our bodies with the necessary nutrients to build and repair bone tissue. In this chapter, we will discuss the best foods to eat for strong bones.

Calcium is the most important nutrient for bone health, and we need to consume adequate amounts of it throughout our lives. The recommended daily intake of calcium for adults is between 1,000 and 1,200 milligrams. Dairy products are the most well-known sources of calcium, but there are also many non-dairy sources. Dark, leafy greens such as kale, collard greens, and spinach are excellent sources of calcium. Other sources include almonds, tofu, sardines, and fortified plant milks.

Vitamin D is essential for calcium absorption and bone health. Our bodies can produce vitamin D when our skin is exposed to sunlight, but many people do not get enough sun exposure or live in areas with limited sunlight. Therefore, it's essential to obtain vitamin D through our diet or supplements. Fatty fish, such as salmon and tuna, are excellent sources of vitamin D. Other sources include egg yolks, mushrooms, and fortified foods.

Magnesium is also necessary for strong bones, as it helps to regulate calcium absorption and supports bone formation. Good sources of magnesium include whole grains, nuts, seeds, legumes, and dark, leafy greens.

Protein is essential for bone health as it provides the building blocks for bone tissue. Good sources of protein include lean meats, poultry, fish, beans, lentils, nuts, and seeds. It's essential to consume a variety of protein sources to ensure you are getting all of the necessary amino acids.

In addition to these nutrients, it's important to limit foods and beverages that can weaken bones. High-sodium diets can increase the amount of calcium lost in the urine, so it's important to limit your sodium intake. Caffeine and alcohol can also weaken bones, so it's best to consume them in moderation.

In conclusion, a diet rich in calcium, vitamin D, magnesium, and protein is essential for strong bones. By including a variety of foods from these groups in your diet and limiting foods and beverages that can weaken bones, you can maintain strong and healthy bones throughout your life.

Chapter 16: Eating for Healthy Skin

Our skin is the largest organ of our body and acts as a barrier to protect us from the environment. It is therefore important to keep it healthy and well-nourished. One way to achieve this is through a balanced diet, as what we eat can have a direct impact on the health of our skin.

Here are some foods that can help promote healthy skin:

Fruits and vegetables: These are rich in antioxidants, vitamins, and minerals that can help protect the skin from damage caused by free radicals. Some examples include berries, oranges, sweet potatoes, leafy greens, and bell peppers.

Omega-3 fatty acids: These healthy fats can help keep the skin moisturized and reduce inflammation, which can lead to a more youthful appearance. Foods rich in omega-3s include fatty fish like salmon, chia seeds, flaxseeds, and walnuts.

Probiotics: These beneficial bacteria can help improve gut health, which in turn can improve the health of the skin. Some examples of probiotic-rich foods include yogurt, kefir, kimchi, and sauerkraut.

Water: Drinking enough water is important for keeping the skin hydrated and preventing dryness and wrinkles. Aim for at least 8 glasses of water per day.

On the other hand, there are also some foods that can have a negative impact on the skin:

Sugar: Consuming too much sugar can lead to inflammation, which can accelerate the aging process and lead to skin problems like acne.

Processed foods: These often contain high amounts of unhealthy fats, sugars, and additives that can lead to skin problems like inflammation and breakouts.

Alcohol: Drinking too much alcohol can dehydrate the skin and lead to inflammation, redness, and premature aging.

In conclusion, a diet that is rich in fruits, vegetables, healthy fats, and probiotics, and low in sugar, processed foods, and alcohol, can help promote healthy and youthful skin. Remember to also stay hydrated by drinking plenty of water throughout the day.

Chapter 17: Eating for a Healthy Heart

Maintaining a healthy heart is essential for overall wellbeing. The food we eat plays a significant role in the health of our heart. Eating a balanced and nutritious diet can help reduce the risk of heart diseases and keep our heart healthy.

Here are some foods that you can incorporate into your diet to maintain a healthy heart:

Fruits and Vegetables: Fruits and vegetables are rich in vitamins, minerals, and fiber, making them an excellent addition to your diet. Eating a variety of colorful fruits and vegetables can help reduce the risk of heart diseases.

Whole Grains: Whole grains, such as oats, barley, and brown rice, are rich in fiber, which helps lower cholesterol levels and reduce the risk of heart diseases. Incorporating whole grains into your diet can help keep your heart healthy.

Lean Protein: Lean protein, such as skinless chicken, fish, and legumes, are excellent sources of protein and are low in saturated fat, making them a healthy addition to your diet.

Healthy Fats: Not all fats are bad for you. Healthy fats, such as monounsaturated and polyunsaturated fats, found in nuts, seeds, avocados, and fatty fish, can help lower cholesterol levels and reduce the risk of heart diseases.

Limit Saturated and Trans Fats: Saturated and trans fats can raise cholesterol levels and increase the risk of heart diseases. Limiting foods high in saturated and trans fats, such as fried foods, processed snacks, and fatty meats, can help keep your heart healthy.

Reduce Sodium: Consuming too much sodium can increase blood pressure, which is a risk factor for heart diseases. Limiting processed foods, canned foods, and adding less salt to your food can help reduce your sodium intake.

Stay Hydrated: Drinking plenty of water can help maintain a healthy heart. Dehydration can lead to an increased heart rate and strain on the heart.

In addition to eating a healthy diet, regular exercise, maintaining a healthy weight, and avoiding smoking can help keep your heart healthy.

Overall, maintaining a healthy heart requires a balanced and nutritious diet, regular exercise, and a healthy lifestyle. Incorporating the foods mentioned above into your diet can help reduce the risk of heart diseases and keep your heart healthy.

Chapter 18: Eating for Weight Loss

One of the most common reasons people turn to healthy eating is to lose weight. While the concept of weight loss may seem straightforward, it can be quite challenging to achieve without the right knowledge and strategies. In this chapter, we will discuss how to eat for weight loss, including what foods to eat and what foods to avoid, as well as helpful tips to make the process easier.

Calories in vs. Calories out

The key to losing weight is to burn more calories than you consume. This means that you need to create a calorie deficit, which can be achieved through a combination of diet and exercise. To determine your daily caloric needs, you can use an online calculator that takes into account your age, gender, height, weight, and activity level.

Focus on Whole, Nutrient-Dense Foods

When it comes to weight loss, not all calories are created equal. Choosing whole, nutrient-dense foods can help you feel fuller for longer periods, and provide your body with the necessary vitamins and minerals. These foods include:

Fruits and vegetables: these low-calorie foods are high in fiber, which can help you feel full and reduce cravings.

Lean protein: such as chicken, fish, tofu, and beans, can help build and repair muscle while keeping you full and satisfied.

Whole grains: such as brown rice, quinoa, and whole wheat bread, are high in fiber, which can help keep you full and provide lasting energy.

Avoid Processed Foods and Sugary Drinks

Processed foods and sugary drinks are high in calories and low in nutrients. They can quickly add up to your daily caloric intake without providing any nutritional value. Instead, choose whole foods and drink plenty of water to stay hydrated.

Watch your Portions

Even healthy foods can lead to weight gain if consumed in excess. One way to control your portions is to use smaller plates, bowls, and cups. Additionally, you can try using the "plate method" by dividing your plate into thirds and filling one-third with lean protein, one-third with non-starchy vegetables, and one-third with whole grains or starchy vegetables.

Eat Mindfully

Eating mindfully means paying attention to your body's hunger and fullness cues, as well as being present and mindful while eating. Try to avoid distractions such as TV or your phone while eating, and take the time to savor your food. This can help prevent overeating and promote mindful eating habits.

Plan Ahead

Planning your meals and snacks ahead of time can help you stay on track and avoid impulsive food choices. Consider meal prepping on weekends or packing healthy snacks to take with you to work or school.

Get Moving

While diet is a crucial component of weight loss, exercise is also essential. Aim for at least 30 minutes of moderate-intensity exercise most days of the week. This can include brisk walking, jogging, cycling, or any other activity that gets your heart rate up.

In summary, eating for weight loss involves creating a calorie deficit by focusing on whole, nutrient-dense foods, avoiding processed foods and sugary drinks, watching your portions, eating mindfully, planning ahead, and incorporating exercise into your daily routine. By following these tips, you can achieve your weight loss goals while also improving your overall health and wellbeing.

Chapter 19: Eating for Muscle Gain

When it comes to building muscle, the right diet is just as important as lifting weights and working out. Eating the right foods in the right amounts can help support muscle growth, repair, and recovery, while also providing the energy and nutrients needed to fuel intense workouts.

Here are some tips for eating to support muscle gain:

Increase your calorie intake: To build muscle, you need to consume more calories than you burn. A calorie surplus provides the energy your body needs to support muscle growth. Aim to consume around 250-500 extra calories per day above your maintenance level.

Eat enough protein: Protein is essential for muscle growth and repair. Aim to consume 1-1.5 grams of protein per pound of bodyweight daily. Good sources of protein include chicken, fish, beef, eggs, dairy, and plant-based options like beans, lentils, tofu, and tempeh.

Include complex carbohydrates: Carbohydrates are the body's primary source of energy. Complex carbs like whole grains, sweet potatoes, and fruits provide a steady release of energy and can help fuel workouts. Aim to consume 2-3 grams of carbs per pound of bodyweight daily.

Don't forget healthy fats: Healthy fats like nuts, seeds, avocado, and olive oil can provide essential fatty acids and help support hormone production. Aim to consume around 0.5-1 gram of fat per pound of bodyweight daily.

Timing is key: To maximize muscle growth, it's important to fuel your body with the right nutrients at the right time. Eat a meal containing protein and carbs within 30 minutes of finishing your workout to support recovery and muscle growth.

Stay hydrated: Drinking enough water is crucial for overall health and performance. Aim to drink at least half your body weight in ounces of water daily. Dehydration can lead to fatigue, cramping, and decreased athletic performance.

Consider supplements: While a well-rounded diet is essential for muscle gain, supplements can also be helpful. Whey protein, creatine, and branched-chain amino acids (BCAAs) are popular choices for supporting muscle growth.

Remember, building muscle takes time and consistency. Eating a diet rich in whole, nutrient-dense foods and maintaining a regular workout routine can help you achieve your muscle gain goals.

Chapter 20: Eating for Better Sleep

Getting a good night's sleep is essential for maintaining a healthy body and mind. Many factors can affect the quality of your sleep, including stress, physical discomfort, and even your diet. Eating the right foods can help promote better sleep and ensure you wake up feeling refreshed and ready for the day ahead. In this chapter, we'll explore some of the best foods to eat for better sleep.

Complex Carbohydrates

Foods high in complex carbohydrates, such as whole grains, fruits, and vegetables, are excellent choices for promoting better sleep. These foods help regulate blood sugar levels, which can prevent spikes and crashes that can disrupt sleep. They also contain fiber, which helps you feel full and satisfied for longer, reducing the likelihood of waking up hungry during the night.

Lean Proteins

Incorporating lean proteins into your diet can help promote better sleep as well. Foods like chicken, fish, and tofu are excellent sources of protein and contain tryptophan, an amino acid that can help increase the production of serotonin, a neurotransmitter that promotes relaxation and sleep. It's essential to choose lean sources of protein to avoid any digestive discomfort that can disrupt sleep.

Nuts and Seeds

Nuts and seeds are a great snack option for those looking to improve their sleep. Almonds, for example, are an excellent source of magnesium, which can help relax muscles and promote a deeper sleep. Walnuts contain melatonin, a hormone that helps regulate the sleep-wake cycle. Chia seeds are another great option, as they contain tryptophan and omega-3 fatty acids, both of which can promote better sleep.

Herbal Teas

Herbal teas can help promote relaxation and calmness before bed, making them an excellent addition to your nighttime routine. Chamomile tea, for example, contains apigenin, an antioxidant that can help reduce inflammation and promote better sleep. Valerian root tea is another popular option, as it can help reduce anxiety and promote relaxation.

Foods to Avoid

While some foods can help promote better sleep, others can have the opposite effect. Avoiding caffeine, alcohol, and sugary foods before bed can help prevent sleep disturbances. Spicy foods can also cause heartburn or indigestion, making it harder to fall asleep.

In conclusion, choosing the right foods can help promote better sleep and ensure you wake up feeling refreshed and energized. Incorporating complex carbohydrates, lean proteins, nuts and seeds, and herbal teas into your diet while avoiding caffeine, alcohol, and sugary foods can help promote a better night's sleep. With a little planning and preparation, you can make sure that what you eat helps you sleep better and feel better.

Chapter 21: Eating for Immune Health

Our immune system plays a vital role in protecting our body against infections, diseases, and illnesses. A strong immune system is crucial for maintaining good health and well-being. While many factors contribute to immune health, including genetics and lifestyle, one of the most important factors is diet. Eating a healthy diet can help boost our immune system, and provide the necessary nutrients that our body needs to function properly.

So, what should we eat for immune health? Here are some of the best foods to include in your diet:

Citrus Fruits

Citrus fruits, such as oranges, grapefruits, and lemons, are rich in vitamin C, which is essential for a healthy immune system. Vitamin C acts as an antioxidant and helps protect our cells from damage. It also helps stimulate the production of white blood cells, which are important for fighting infections.

Garlic

Garlic is a powerful antioxidant and has antimicrobial properties that help boost the immune system. It is also rich in sulfur compounds, which help improve the function of white blood cells.

Ginger

Ginger is a popular spice that has been used for its medicinal properties for centuries. It has anti-inflammatory and antioxidant properties, which help reduce inflammation in the body and boost the immune system.

Yogurt

Yogurt is a great source of probiotics, which are beneficial bacteria that live in our gut. Probiotics help strengthen the immune system by improving the function of our gut microbiome, which plays a critical role in immune function.

Leafy Greens

Leafy greens, such as spinach, kale, and broccoli, are rich in vitamins and minerals, including vitamin C, vitamin E, and antioxidants. These nutrients help protect our cells from damage and support the immune system.

Nuts and Seeds

Nuts and seeds, such as almonds, walnuts, and sunflower seeds, are rich in healthy fats, vitamins, and minerals. They also contain antioxidants and anti-inflammatory compounds, which help support immune health.

Turmeric

Turmeric is a spice that has been used for its medicinal properties for centuries. It contains curcumin, which has powerful antioxidant and anti-inflammatory properties that help boost the immune system.

In addition to including these foods in your diet, it's important to avoid processed foods, sugar, and excessive alcohol consumption, as these can weaken the immune system. It's also important to stay hydrated and to get enough sleep, as both of these factors also play a critical role in immune function.

In conclusion, eating a healthy diet that includes a variety of immune-boosting foods can help strengthen our immune system, and protect us against infections and illnesses. By making simple changes to our diet and lifestyle, we can support our immune health and enjoy a lifetime of good health and well-being.

Chapter 22: Eating for Gut Health

Maintaining gut health is crucial for overall well-being as the gut plays an essential role in our immune system, digestion, and nutrient absorption. The key to having a healthy gut is to maintain a balance of good bacteria in the digestive tract. Diet plays a significant role in achieving this balance, and here are some tips on how to eat for gut health.

Focus on Fiber-rich Foods

Fiber is essential for a healthy gut, as it feeds the good bacteria in our digestive tract. A diet high in fiber can promote regular bowel movements, prevent constipation, and reduce the risk of digestive disorders such as irritable bowel syndrome (IBS) and diverticulitis. Some good sources of fiber include whole grains, fruits, vegetables, legumes, nuts, and seeds.

Include Fermented Foods

Fermented foods are rich in probiotics, which are beneficial bacteria that help to maintain a healthy gut. Some examples of fermented foods include yogurt, kefir, kimchi, sauerkraut, miso, and tempeh. When selecting fermented foods, look for those that are minimally processed and do not contain added sugars.

Reduce Intake of Processed Foods

Processed foods are often low in fiber and high in sugar and unhealthy fats, which can disrupt the balance of good bacteria in the gut. It's best to limit your intake of processed foods and opt for whole, nutrient-dense foods instead. Eating a variety of colorful fruits and vegetables, lean proteins, and healthy fats can help to support a healthy gut.

Stay Hydrated

Drinking plenty of water is essential for maintaining a healthy gut. Water helps to flush out waste products and toxins from the body and prevents constipation. Aim to drink at least eight glasses of water a day, and if you struggle to drink enough water, try infusing it with fruits or herbs for a refreshing flavor.

Limit Alcohol and Caffeine

Excessive intake of alcohol and caffeine can disrupt the balance of good bacteria in the gut and contribute to digestive issues such as bloating, constipation, and diarrhea. It's best to limit your intake of these substances and opt for water or herbal teas instead.

Take Probiotic Supplements

If you struggle to include enough fermented foods in your diet, taking a probiotic supplement can help to boost the levels of good bacteria in your gut. When selecting a probiotic supplement, look for one that contains a variety of strains of beneficial bacteria and is shelf-stable.

In conclusion, maintaining a healthy gut is essential for overall health and well-being. By focusing on fiber-rich foods, including fermented foods in your diet, limiting processed foods, staying hydrated, limiting alcohol and caffeine intake, and taking probiotic supplements, you can support a healthy gut and reduce the risk of digestive disorders.

Chapter 23: Eating for Brain Health

When we think about healthy foods, we often focus on how they can benefit our physical health. However, what we eat also has a significant impact on our brain health. Just like the rest of our body, our brain requires certain nutrients to function properly, and what we eat can either support or harm our cognitive health. In this chapter, we'll explore some of the best foods for brain health and why they're important.

Omega-3 Fatty Acids:

Omega-3 fatty acids are one of the most important nutrients for brain health. They're essential for the development and maintenance of the brain and play a crucial role in cognitive function. Omega-3s are found in fatty fish like salmon, sardines, and mackerel, as well as in plant-based sources like chia seeds, flaxseed, and walnuts. Eating these foods regularly can improve memory and cognitive function and reduce the risk of cognitive decline and dementia.

Antioxidants:

Antioxidants are compounds that protect our cells from damage caused by free radicals. They're found in many fruits and vegetables, including berries, leafy greens, and cruciferous vegetables like broccoli and cauliflower. Antioxidants have been linked to improved cognitive function and a reduced risk of Alzheimer's disease.

Whole Grains:

Whole grains are an excellent source of complex carbohydrates, which are the primary source of energy for the brain. They also contain B vitamins, which are essential for brain health. Eating whole grains like oatmeal, quinoa, and brown rice can improve memory and cognitive function.

Water:

Water is essential for all bodily functions, including brain function. Even mild dehydration can impair cognitive performance, so it's important to drink plenty of water throughout the day. Drinking water can also improve mood and reduce fatigue.

Nuts:

Nuts are a great source of healthy fats, protein, and fiber, as well as a range of micronutrients that are important for brain health, such as vitamin E, magnesium, and selenium. Eating nuts like almonds, cashews, and peanuts can improve cognitive function and reduce the risk of cognitive decline.

Conclusion:

Eating for brain health is just as important as eating for physical health. By including foods like fatty fish, berries, whole grains, and nuts in your diet, you can support cognitive function, reduce the risk of cognitive decline, and improve overall brain health. Remember to also stay hydrated by drinking plenty of water throughout the day. Making these changes to your diet can help you feel sharper, more alert, and more focused, which can improve your overall quality of life.

Chapter 24: Eating for Longevity

When it comes to healthy eating, there is one goal that many people share: to live a long and healthy life. While genetics certainly play a role in determining our lifespan, there are many lifestyle factors that we can control, including our diet. Eating for longevity means choosing foods that support our overall health and reduce our risk of chronic diseases.

One of the key components of a longevity-promoting diet is a focus on whole, minimally processed foods. These include fruits, vegetables, whole grains, legumes, nuts, and seeds. These foods are rich in a variety of nutrients that support optimal health, including fiber, vitamins, minerals, and antioxidants.

Fiber is especially important for longevity, as it helps to promote healthy digestion and reduce inflammation in the body. Inflammation is a key factor in many chronic diseases, including heart disease, diabetes, and cancer. By eating a diet rich in fiber, we can help to reduce our risk of these conditions.

Another important component of a longevity-promoting diet is the inclusion of healthy fats. Omega-3 fatty acids, found in fatty fish like salmon, as well as in nuts and seeds, have been shown to reduce inflammation and improve heart health. Monounsaturated and polyunsaturated fats, found in foods like avocados, olive oil, and nuts, can also help to support healthy cholesterol levels and reduce the risk of heart disease.

In addition to including these key nutrients, a longevity-promoting diet also means limiting or avoiding foods that are known to be harmful to our health. Processed foods, refined sugars, and trans fats should be avoided whenever possible, as they have been linked to a variety of chronic health conditions.

Another important aspect of a longevity-promoting diet is portion control. Overeating, even of healthy foods, can lead to weight gain and increased risk of chronic diseases. By listening to our bodies and eating until we are satisfied, rather than overly full, we can help to support our health and reduce our risk of disease.

Finally, it's important to remember that healthy eating is just one part of a healthy lifestyle. Regular exercise, stress management, and getting enough sleep are also important for promoting longevity and optimal health.

In conclusion, eating for longevity means choosing whole, minimally processed foods that are rich in fiber, healthy fats, and a variety of nutrients. It also means limiting or avoiding foods that are known to be harmful to our health and practicing portion control. By combining healthy eating with other lifestyle factors, we can help to promote optimal health and increase our chances of living a long and healthy life.

Chapter 25: The Benefits of Organic Foods

Organic foods are those that are produced using environmentally and animal-friendly farming practices, without the use of synthetic pesticides, fertilizers, or genetically modified organisms (GMOs). These foods are grown using natural methods that prioritize soil health, biodiversity, and sustainability.

There are many benefits of consuming organic foods, both for our own health and for the environment. Here are just a few of the reasons why organic foods are a great choice for anyone looking to improve their diet:

Reduced exposure to harmful chemicals

Organic farming practices avoid the use of synthetic pesticides and fertilizers, which can be harmful to human health. These chemicals have been linked to a range of health problems, including cancer, reproductive issues, and neurological disorders. By choosing organic foods, you can reduce your exposure to these harmful chemicals.

Higher nutrient content

Organic foods have been shown to have higher nutrient content than conventionally grown foods. This is because organic farming practices focus on building healthy soil, which in turn leads to healthier, more nutrient-dense crops. For example, studies have shown that organic fruits and vegetables can contain up to 40% more antioxidants than conventionally grown varieties.

Better for the environment

Organic farming practices are designed to be more sustainable and environmentally friendly than conventional farming practices. Organic farmers use techniques like crop rotation, cover cropping, and composting to build healthy soil and reduce the use of synthetic inputs. This helps to protect soil health, preserve biodiversity, and reduce pollution.

Better for animal welfare

Organic farming practices also prioritize animal welfare. Organic livestock are raised in more humane conditions than conventionally raised animals, with access to pasture and a diet free of antibiotics and growth hormones. This leads to healthier, happier animals, and can also result in higher quality meat and dairy products.

Better taste

Many people find that organic foods taste better than conventionally grown foods. This may be because organic crops are grown in healthier soil, which can lead to more flavorful, aromatic produce. Additionally, organic farmers often focus on growing heirloom varieties of fruits and vegetables, which may have unique and interesting flavors.

Overall, there are many benefits to choosing organic foods for your diet. By prioritizing your health, the health of the environment, and the welfare of animals, you can make a positive impact on the world around you while also enjoying delicious, nutrient-dense foods.

Chapter 26: The Benefits of Seasonal Eating

Eating seasonal foods has been a way of life for humans for thousands of years. However, with the modern availability of food from all over the world, seasonal eating has become less common. Nevertheless, there are many benefits to eating seasonal foods that go beyond simply enjoying the freshest and most flavorful produce. In this chapter, we will explore the benefits of seasonal eating and how it can contribute to a healthy lifestyle.

Nutritional Benefits

Eating seasonally means that you are consuming fruits and vegetables when they are at their peak in terms of nutrition. For example, tomatoes are at their most nutritious in the summer when they are fully ripened by the sun. Consuming these nutrient-dense foods at the right time can help you get more vitamins, minerals, and antioxidants that your body needs to function properly.

Environmental Benefits

Seasonal eating also has a positive impact on the environment. When you choose to eat seasonal produce, you are supporting local farmers and reducing the carbon footprint associated with transporting food over long distances. Additionally, seasonal produce is grown in its natural environment and requires less energy to produce, which means that it has a lower environmental impact than produce that is grown in greenhouses or shipped from other countries.

Economic Benefits

Eating seasonally can also be a cost-effective way to shop for groceries. When fruits and vegetables are in season, there is often an abundance of them, which drives prices down. In contrast, when produce is out of season, it can be more expensive to transport and store, which leads to higher prices for consumers. By eating seasonally, you can save money on your grocery bill and support local farmers at the same time.

Variety

Eating seasonally can also introduce more variety into your diet. When you eat the same fruits and vegetables year-round, it can become boring and repetitive. However, when you eat seasonally, you are exposed to a wider range of fruits and vegetables, which can help you get more variety in your diet. This, in turn, can help you get a wider range of nutrients that your body needs to stay healthy.

Taste and Flavor

Finally, eating seasonally means that you are consuming produce that is at its peak in terms of taste and flavor. Fruits and vegetables that are in season are often picked at the right time, which means that they are sweeter, juicier, and more flavorful than produce that is picked before it is fully ripened. By eating seasonally, you can enjoy the full range of flavors that nature has to offer.

In conclusion, there are many benefits to eating seasonally, including nutritional benefits, environmental benefits, economic benefits, variety, and taste. By choosing to eat seasonal produce, you can improve your overall health and well-being while supporting local farmers and reducing your environmental impact. So next time you go grocery shopping, try to choose fruits and vegetables that are in season and enjoy the full range of flavors that nature has to offer.

Chapter 27: The Benefits of Eating Local

Eating local is becoming an increasingly popular trend, and for good reason. Not only is it better for the environment and the local economy, but it can also have numerous benefits for your health. In this chapter, we will explore the various benefits of eating local and how it can help you maintain a healthy diet.

Nutrient-Dense Foods

When you eat local, you are more likely to consume fresh, nutrient-dense foods. This is because local foods are often picked at peak ripeness and delivered to local markets or restaurants quickly, ensuring that they retain more of their vitamins and minerals. Additionally, local farmers tend to focus on growing a variety of fruits and vegetables, which can provide you with a range of nutrients that you may not get from imported foods.

Lower in Chemicals

One of the biggest benefits of eating local is that you are more likely to consume foods that are free of harmful chemicals. Local farmers tend to use fewer pesticides and herbicides than large-scale producers, which means that their crops are less likely to be contaminated with harmful chemicals. Additionally, local farmers tend to use organic methods and natural fertilizers, which can help to preserve soil health and reduce the risk of chemical runoff into local water sources.

Supports Local Economy

When you eat local, you are not only benefiting your health, but you are also supporting the local economy.

Local farmers, producers, and businesses rely on community support to stay in business, and every dollar you spend on local foods helps to stimulate the local economy. This can have a ripple effect, as the money you spend locally will circulate within the community and support other businesses.

Seasonal Eating

Eating local can also encourage you to eat seasonally. When you buy foods that are in season, they are more likely to be fresh and nutrient-dense, as they have not been shipped long distances or stored for long periods of time. Additionally, seasonal eating can help to diversify your diet and encourage you to try new fruits and vegetables that you may not have tried before.

Environmental Benefits

Finally, eating local has numerous environmental benefits. When you buy foods that are grown or produced locally, you are reducing the carbon footprint associated with transportation and storage. Additionally, local farmers tend to use sustainable and environmentally-friendly methods, which can help to preserve soil health, reduce water usage, and promote biodiversity.

In conclusion, eating local can have numerous benefits for your health, the environment, and the local economy. By consuming fresh, nutrient-dense foods that are free of harmful chemicals, you can help to support the health of your body and the planet. Additionally, by supporting local farmers and businesses, you can help to build a strong and vibrant community. So the next time you're at the market or dining out, consider choosing local options for a healthier and more sustainable lifestyle.

Chapter 28: The Benefits of Plant-Based Diets

Plant-based diets have been gaining popularity in recent years, and for good reason. Not only are these diets rich in nutrients and vitamins, but they also offer a variety of health benefits. In this chapter, we will explore some of the benefits of plant-based diets.

Lower Risk of Chronic Diseases

Studies have shown that plant-based diets are associated with a lower risk of chronic diseases such as heart disease, diabetes, and certain cancers. This is because plant-based diets are typically high in fiber, vitamins, and antioxidants, all of which are known to promote good health. In addition, plant-based diets are generally low in saturated fat and cholesterol, which are both known to increase the risk of chronic diseases.

Improved Digestive Health

Plant-based diets are rich in fiber, which can improve digestive health. Fiber promotes regular bowel movements, reduces constipation, and can prevent certain types of digestive disorders. In addition, plant-based diets are generally low in processed foods, which are known to cause digestive issues such as bloating and gas.

Weight Management

Plant-based diets are generally lower in calories and higher in fiber than animal-based diets. This makes it easier to manage weight and maintain a healthy body weight. In addition, plant-based diets are typically more satiating, which means that people tend to eat less and feel fuller for longer periods of time.

Improved Mental Health

Studies have shown that plant-based diets may improve mental health. For example, a study published in the journal Nutritional Neuroscience found that people who followed a plant-based diet had lower levels of anxiety and depression than those who followed an omnivorous diet. This may be because plant-based diets are rich in nutrients such as vitamins B6 and B12, which are known to promote good mental health.

Environmental Benefits

Plant-based diets are also better for the environment than animal-based diets. Livestock production is a major contributor to greenhouse gas emissions, deforestation, and water pollution. By choosing to eat a plant-based diet, individuals can reduce their carbon footprint and help protect the planet.

In conclusion, plant-based diets offer a wide range of health benefits, including a lower risk of chronic diseases, improved digestive health, weight management, improved mental health, and environmental benefits. By incorporating more plant-based foods into your diet, you can improve your health and help protect the planet.

Chapter 29: The Benefits of Fermented Foods

Fermented foods have been consumed by people for thousands of years, with many cultures around the world having their own traditional fermented foods. In recent years, fermented foods have gained popularity in the health and wellness community, with many touting the numerous health benefits associated with their consumption. In this chapter, we will explore the benefits of fermented foods and why they should be included in a healthy diet.

Improved Digestion

One of the most well-known benefits of fermented foods is their ability to improve digestion. Fermentation is a process that involves the breakdown of carbohydrates and proteins in foods by beneficial bacteria, yeast, and other microorganisms. This process produces enzymes that help break down food and make it easier for our bodies to digest. Additionally, fermented foods contain probiotics, which are live bacteria and yeasts that are beneficial for our gut microbiome. These probiotics can help improve digestion by aiding in the breakdown and absorption of nutrients, reducing inflammation, and supporting immune function.

Enhanced Nutrient Absorption

Fermented foods not only aid in digestion, but they can also help enhance nutrient absorption. The fermentation process breaks down food into more easily digestible forms, making it easier for the body to absorb nutrients. For example, fermented dairy products such as yogurt and kefir are easier to digest than regular milk, and the fermentation process increases the bioavailability of calcium and other nutrients.

Boosted Immune System

Consuming fermented foods can also help boost the immune system. The gut microbiome plays an essential role in immune function, and a healthy gut microbiome can help protect against infections, reduce inflammation, and support overall immune health. Fermented foods contain probiotics that can help support a healthy gut microbiome and promote immune function.

Improved Mental Health

Recent research has also shown that consuming fermented foods can have a positive impact on mental health. The gut-brain connection is a complex system, and the gut microbiome plays a crucial role in regulating mood and mental health. Studies have found that consuming fermented foods can help improve mood, reduce anxiety, and even alleviate symptoms of depression.

Increased Diversity in the Gut Microbiome

The gut microbiome is a complex ecosystem of microorganisms that live in our digestive tract. A healthy gut microbiome is diverse, with many different types of bacteria and other microorganisms living in harmony. Consuming fermented foods can help increase the diversity of the gut microbiome by introducing new strains of beneficial bacteria and supporting their growth.

In conclusion, fermented foods are a valuable addition to a healthy diet. They offer numerous benefits, including improved digestion, enhanced nutrient absorption, boosted immune function, improved mental health, and increased diversity in the gut microbiome. Adding fermented foods such as yogurt, kimchi, sauerkraut, and kefir to your diet can provide you with a range of health benefits, and they are delicious too!

Chapter 30: The Benefits of Whole Foods

Whole foods refer to foods that are minimally processed and are as close to their natural state as possible. These foods are often unrefined and are free from additives, preservatives, and other chemicals. They include fruits, vegetables, whole grains, nuts, seeds, and legumes. In this chapter, we will explore the benefits of whole foods and how they can contribute to a healthy diet.

Nutrient-rich: Whole foods are packed with essential nutrients, including vitamins, minerals, fiber, and antioxidants. These nutrients are important for maintaining good health, and they are often lost during the processing of food. By eating whole foods, you can ensure that you are getting all of the nutrients your body needs to function at its best.

Improved digestion: Whole foods are rich in fiber, which can help improve digestion and prevent constipation. Fiber is also essential for maintaining healthy gut bacteria, which can improve overall gut health and reduce the risk of digestive disorders.

Reduced inflammation: Many whole foods, such as fruits, vegetables, and nuts, contain anti-inflammatory compounds that can help reduce inflammation in the body. Chronic inflammation has been linked to numerous health problems, including heart disease, cancer, and autoimmune disorders.

Weight management: Whole foods are often lower in calories and higher in fiber than processed foods, which can help with weight management. The fiber in whole foods helps you feel full for longer, reducing the urge to overeat or snack on unhealthy foods.

Improved heart health: Whole foods, especially those high in fiber, can help improve heart health by lowering cholesterol levels, reducing blood pressure, and improving blood sugar control. This can reduce the risk of heart disease, stroke, and other cardiovascular problems.

Reduced risk of chronic diseases: Eating a diet rich in whole foods has been linked to a reduced risk of chronic diseases, such as type 2 diabetes, cancer, and Alzheimer's disease. The nutrients and compounds found in whole foods have numerous health benefits that can help protect against these diseases.

Sustainable and ethical: Whole foods are often grown using sustainable farming practices, which are better for the environment and can help reduce your carbon footprint. Additionally, buying whole foods from local farmers and producers can support the local economy and promote ethical food production.

In conclusion, incorporating whole foods into your diet can provide numerous health benefits, including improved digestion, reduced inflammation, weight management, improved heart health, and a reduced risk of chronic diseases. By choosing whole foods, you can ensure that you are getting all of the nutrients your body needs while supporting sustainable and ethical food production practices.

Chapter 31: The Benefits of Superfoods

Superfoods are nutrient-dense foods that offer a wide range of health benefits. They are packed with vitamins, minerals, antioxidants, and other essential nutrients that our body needs to function properly. Incorporating these foods into your diet can help you maintain a healthy weight, reduce your risk of chronic diseases, and improve your overall well-being. Here are some of the benefits of superfoods:

Nutrient-rich: Superfoods are packed with nutrients that are essential for good health. They are a great source of vitamins, minerals, and antioxidants that are important for maintaining healthy skin, hair, and nails. They also help to boost the immune system and reduce inflammation in the body.

Weight management: Superfoods are low in calories but high in nutrients, making them a great addition to any weight management plan. They help to fill you up without adding excess calories, which can help you to eat less and feel more satisfied.

Heart health: Superfoods are great for your heart. They are rich in heart-healthy nutrients like omega-3 fatty acids, fiber, and antioxidants, which can help to reduce your risk of heart disease. They also help to lower your blood pressure and cholesterol levels.

Digestive health: Superfoods are rich in fiber, which is essential for good digestive health. They help to keep your digestive system functioning properly and can help to prevent constipation, diarrhea, and other digestive problems.

Brain health: Superfoods are also good for your brain. They are rich in nutrients that can help to improve cognitive function and memory. They also help to reduce your risk of age-related cognitive decline and dementia.

Energy and vitality: Superfoods can help to boost your energy levels and improve your overall vitality. They provide your body with the nutrients it needs to function properly, which can help to reduce fatigue and improve your mood.

Some examples of superfoods include:

Berries: Blueberries, strawberries, raspberries, and other berries are packed with antioxidants and other essential nutrients.

Leafy greens: Spinach, kale, and other leafy greens are a great source of vitamins and minerals, including iron, calcium, and vitamin C.

Nuts and seeds: Almonds, walnuts, chia seeds, and flaxseeds are rich in omega-3 fatty acids and other essential nutrients.

Whole grains: Whole grains like brown rice, quinoa, and oats are a great source of fiber and other essential nutrients.

Fish: Salmon, tuna, and other fatty fish are rich in omega-3 fatty acids, which are essential for good heart and brain health.

In conclusion, superfoods are a great addition to any healthy diet. They are nutrient-dense foods that offer a wide range of health benefits, including weight management, heart health, digestive health, brain health, and more. By incorporating these foods into your diet, you can improve your overall health and well-being.

Chapter 32: The Benefits of Nuts and Seeds

Nuts and seeds are nutrient-dense foods that provide a wide range of health benefits. They are an excellent source of healthy fats, fiber, protein, vitamins, and minerals. Incorporating nuts and seeds into your diet can help reduce the risk of chronic diseases such as heart disease, diabetes, and cancer. Here are some of the benefits of nuts and seeds:

Promotes Heart Health

Nuts and seeds are rich in heart-healthy monounsaturated and polyunsaturated fats. These fats help to lower LDL (bad) cholesterol levels and increase HDL (good) cholesterol levels. They also contain antioxidants that help to reduce inflammation, which is a major risk factor for heart disease.

Helps with Weight Management

Although nuts and seeds are high in calories, they are also very filling. Studies have shown that adding nuts and seeds to your diet can help you feel more satisfied and reduce your overall calorie intake. This can lead to weight loss and improved weight management.

Reduces Inflammation

Nuts and seeds are rich in antioxidants and anti-inflammatory compounds, such as omega-3 fatty acids, magnesium, and vitamin E. These nutrients help to reduce inflammation throughout the body, which is linked to many chronic diseases.

Lowers Blood Sugar Levels

Nuts and seeds have a low glycemic index, meaning they don't cause a rapid spike in blood sugar levels. This is particularly beneficial for people with diabetes or those at risk of developing diabetes.

Boosts Brain Function

Nuts and seeds are high in healthy fats, such as omega-3 fatty acids, which are essential for brain function. Studies have shown that consuming nuts and seeds regularly can improve cognitive function and reduce the risk of neurodegenerative diseases such as Alzheimer's.

Improves Bone Health

Nuts and seeds are rich in calcium, magnesium, and phosphorus, which are essential for strong bones. Studies have shown that consuming nuts and seeds regularly can help to improve bone density and reduce the risk of osteoporosis.

Helps with Digestion

Nuts and seeds are high in fiber, which is essential for healthy digestion. Fiber helps to keep you feeling full, promotes bowel regularity, and supports the growth of healthy gut bacteria.

In conclusion, nuts and seeds are an excellent addition to any healthy diet. They provide a wide range of health benefits, including promoting heart health, reducing inflammation, boosting brain function, improving bone health, and aiding in digestion. Incorporating nuts and seeds into your diet can be as simple as adding them to your breakfast, snacking on them throughout the day, or using them as a topping for salads and other dishes. So why not start adding them to your diet today and reap the many benefits they have to offer?

Chapter 33: The Benefits of Berries

Berries are among the most beloved fruits worldwide, and they are celebrated not only for their delicious taste but also for their numerous health benefits. Berries come in many shapes, sizes, and colors, but what they have in common is that they are all packed with essential vitamins, minerals, and antioxidants that are vital to our health.

One of the most significant benefits of berries is their high antioxidant content. Antioxidants are molecules that protect our cells from damage caused by free radicals, which are unstable molecules that can cause cellular damage and contribute to the development of chronic diseases like cancer, diabetes, and heart disease. Berries are particularly high in antioxidants, and some studies have shown that they may have up to ten times the antioxidant activity of other fruits and vegetables. This means that incorporating berries into your diet may help to reduce inflammation and improve overall health.

Another benefit of berries is their high fiber content. Fiber is an essential nutrient that helps to regulate digestion and maintain a healthy gut. Berries are particularly high in soluble fiber, which is the type of fiber that dissolves in water and forms a gel-like substance in the gut. This type of fiber helps to slow down the absorption of sugar and can help to lower cholesterol levels.

Berries are also an excellent source of vitamins and minerals. For example, strawberries are high in vitamin C, which is essential for immune function and collagen production. Blueberries are high in vitamin K, which is important for blood clotting, and raspberries are high in manganese, which is essential for bone health. Incorporating a variety of berries into your diet can help to ensure that you are getting a wide range of essential nutrients.

Finally, berries are a low-calorie, nutrient-dense food, making them an excellent addition to any diet. Unlike processed foods and sugary snacks, which can be high in calories and low in nutrients, berries offer a delicious and healthy way to satisfy your sweet tooth. They are also easy to incorporate into your diet and can be enjoyed fresh, frozen, or dried.

In conclusion, berries are a delicious and healthy food that offers numerous health benefits. They are high in antioxidants, fiber, vitamins, and minerals and can help to reduce inflammation, regulate digestion, and support overall health. Whether you enjoy them as a snack, a topping for your breakfast cereal, or as an ingredient in your favorite recipe, incorporating berries into your diet is an excellent way to promote optimal health and wellness.

Chapter 34: The Benefits of Leafy Greens

Leafy greens, which are vegetables that have edible leaves, are some of the most nutritious foods that you can consume. They are packed with a variety of vitamins, minerals, and other nutrients that are essential for good health.

One of the primary benefits of leafy greens is their high nutrient content. They are an excellent source of vitamin K, which is essential for proper blood clotting and bone health. They also contain significant amounts of vitamin A, vitamin C, and folate, all of which are important for maintaining healthy skin, eyes, and immune system.

Leafy greens are also rich in antioxidants, which can help to protect your cells from damage caused by free radicals. This can lower your risk of developing chronic diseases, such as cancer, heart disease, and Alzheimer's disease.

Eating leafy greens can also help you to maintain a healthy weight. They are low in calories and high in fiber, which can help you to feel full and satisfied after eating. This can make it easier to stick to a healthy diet and avoid overeating.

Additionally, leafy greens are an excellent source of plant-based protein, which is important for building and repairing muscles. They also contain a variety of other nutrients, such as iron, calcium, and magnesium, that are essential for good health.

Some of the most common types of leafy greens include spinach, kale, collard greens, and arugula. These vegetables can be eaten raw in salads, added to smoothies, or cooked in a variety of dishes. They can also be used as a substitute for other types of greens in recipes.

Overall, incorporating more leafy greens into your diet can provide a wide range of health benefits. They are nutritious, low in calories, and can help to reduce your risk of developing chronic diseases. So if you want to improve your health and well-being, be sure to include plenty of leafy greens in your diet.

Chapter 35: The Benefits of Cruciferous Vegetables

Cruciferous vegetables are a group of vegetables that are

renowned for their numerous health benefits. These vegetables are packed with essential vitamins, minerals, and antioxidants that promote good health and help prevent chronic diseases. Here are some of the benefits of cruciferous vegetables:

Protection against Cancer: Cruciferous vegetables are rich in compounds known as glucosinolates, which are broken down in the body to form indoles and isothiocyanates. These compounds have been shown to inhibit the growth of cancer cells and reduce the risk of developing several types of cancers, including lung, breast, prostate, and colon cancer.

Anti-Inflammatory Properties: Cruciferous vegetables are high in antioxidants such as vitamins C, E, and beta-carotene. These antioxidants help to neutralize free radicals, which are harmful molecules that cause inflammation and damage to cells. By reducing inflammation, cruciferous vegetables can help to prevent chronic diseases such as heart disease, arthritis, and diabetes.

Improved Digestive Health: Cruciferous vegetables are rich in fiber, which is essential for maintaining healthy digestion. Fiber helps to regulate bowel movements and prevent constipation, and it also feeds the beneficial bacteria in the gut. Eating cruciferous vegetables regularly can help to maintain a healthy gut microbiome, which is essential for overall health.

Reduced Risk of Cardiovascular Disease: Cruciferous vegetables are rich in nutrients such as folate, potassium, and magnesium, which are essential for heart health. Studies have shown that eating cruciferous vegetables can help to lower blood pressure and cholesterol levels, reducing the risk of cardiovascular disease.

Better Bone Health: Cruciferous vegetables are a good source of calcium, which is essential for healthy bones. They also contain other nutrients such as vitamin K and magnesium, which are important for bone health. Eating cruciferous vegetables regularly can help to reduce the risk of osteoporosis and fractures.

Some examples of cruciferous vegetables include broccoli, cauliflower, cabbage, Brussels sprouts, kale, and bok choy. These vegetables can be eaten raw or cooked, and they can be added to salads, stir-fries, soups, and stews. To get the most benefit from cruciferous vegetables, it is best to eat a variety of them regularly.

In conclusion, cruciferous vegetables are a powerhouse of nutrition that can provide numerous health benefits. Eating these vegetables regularly can help to protect against cancer, reduce inflammation, improve digestive health, lower the risk of cardiovascular disease, and promote better bone health. So, make sure to add these nutritious vegetables to your diet for optimal health and wellbeing.

Chapter 36: The Benefits of Root Vegetables

Root vegetables are some of the most nutrient-dense foods available, making them an excellent addition to any healthy diet. These vegetables are rich in vitamins, minerals, fiber, and antioxidants that can help improve overall health and prevent chronic diseases.

One of the main benefits of root vegetables is their high fiber content. Fiber is essential for maintaining healthy digestion, regulating blood sugar levels, and promoting feelings of fullness, which can help with weight management. Many root vegetables, such as sweet potatoes and beets, are also low on the glycemic index, meaning they have a minimal effect on blood sugar levels.

Root vegetables are also an excellent source of vitamins and minerals. Sweet potatoes, for example, are loaded with vitamin A, which is essential for maintaining healthy vision, skin, and immune function. Carrots are another root vegetable that is rich in vitamin A, as well as other important nutrients such as vitamin K and potassium.

Beets, another popular root vegetable, are high in antioxidants called betalains, which give them their vibrant color. These antioxidants can help protect against oxidative stress and inflammation, which are associated with many chronic diseases, including cancer, heart disease, and Alzheimer's disease.

Other root vegetables, such as turnips, parsnips, and rutabagas, are also rich in vitamins and minerals. Turnips are a good source of vitamin C, while parsnips are high in folate, a B vitamin that is important for brain health. Rutabagas, on the other hand, are an excellent source of potassium, which can help lower blood pressure and reduce the risk of heart disease.

In addition to their nutritional benefits, root vegetables are versatile and can be used in a variety of dishes. They can be roasted, mashed, sautéed, or added to soups and stews, making them an easy addition to any meal.

Overall, incorporating root vegetables into your diet is an excellent way to boost your nutrient intake and improve your overall health. These delicious and versatile vegetables offer a range of benefits that can help reduce the risk of chronic diseases and promote overall well-being.

Chapter 37: The Benefits of Legumes

Legumes are a type of plant-based food that has been consumed by humans for thousands of years. They include a variety of beans, lentils, chickpeas, and peas. Legumes are not only affordable and easy to prepare, but they also provide a wide range of health benefits. In this chapter, we will explore the many ways that legumes can contribute to a healthy diet.

High in Nutrients

Legumes are a great source of essential nutrients, including fiber, protein, complex carbohydrates, iron, and folate. They are also rich in vitamins and minerals such as potassium, magnesium, and zinc. In fact, some studies suggest that legumes are one of the most nutrient-dense foods available.

Good for Digestive Health

Legumes are high in fiber, which is essential for good digestive health. Fiber can help regulate bowel movements, prevent constipation, and promote the growth of healthy gut bacteria. Eating legumes regularly can also reduce the risk of certain digestive disorders such as diverticulitis and inflammatory bowel disease.

Help Manage Blood Sugar

Legumes are a low glycemic index food, meaning they do not cause rapid spikes in blood sugar levels. This makes them an ideal food for people with diabetes or those at risk of developing the disease. Eating legumes regularly may also improve insulin sensitivity and reduce the risk of developing type 2 diabetes.

Reduce Risk of Heart Disease

Legumes are a great source of heart-healthy nutrients such as fiber, potassium, and magnesium. Studies have shown that eating legumes regularly can help lower blood pressure, reduce cholesterol levels, and decrease the risk of heart disease. One study even found that consuming legumes can reduce the risk of coronary heart disease by up to 11%.

Support Weight Loss

Legumes are a low-fat, low-calorie food that can help support weight loss. They are high in fiber and protein, which can help reduce appetite and keep you feeling full for longer periods. Some studies suggest that incorporating legumes into your diet may help reduce body weight, body mass index (BMI), and waist circumference.

In conclusion, legumes are a versatile, affordable, and nutrient-rich food that can offer a range of health benefits. Whether you are looking to improve digestive health, manage blood sugar levels, reduce the risk of heart disease, or support weight loss, adding legumes to your diet can help you achieve your goals. So, next time you are at the grocery store, be sure to pick up a few cans or bags of your favorite legumes and start reaping the benefits.

Chapter 38: The Benefits of Whole Grains

Whole grains are an important part of a healthy diet, and they offer a wide range of benefits for our overall health and well-being. Unlike refined grains, which have been processed to remove the bran and germ, whole grains are left intact, providing us with essential nutrients and fiber that are necessary for good health.

One of the primary benefits of consuming whole grains is their high fiber content. Fiber is an essential nutrient that helps to regulate our digestion and keep our digestive system healthy. It also helps to reduce our risk of developing chronic diseases such as heart disease, diabetes, and certain types of cancer. Whole grains are particularly rich in a type of fiber called insoluble fiber, which helps to move food through our digestive system and promotes regular bowel movements.

Whole grains are also a good source of important vitamins and minerals, including B vitamins, iron, zinc, and magnesium. These nutrients are essential for a wide range of bodily functions, from maintaining healthy bones and teeth to supporting the immune system and promoting healthy brain function. By consuming whole grains as part of a balanced diet, we can ensure that we are getting the nutrients our bodies need to function at their best.

Another benefit of whole grains is their low glycemic index, which means that they are digested slowly and do not cause a rapid spike in blood sugar levels. This makes them an ideal food choice for people with diabetes or those at risk of developing the condition. Additionally, whole grains can help to reduce our risk of heart disease by lowering cholesterol levels and improving blood pressure.

Incorporating whole grains into our diet is relatively easy, as they are widely available and can be found in a variety of forms, including whole wheat bread, brown rice, oatmeal, quinoa, and barley. When choosing whole grain products, it's important to read the label carefully to ensure that they are truly whole grain and not just refined grains that have been colored to appear whole. Look for products that list whole grains as the first ingredient and avoid those that contain added sugars or other additives.

In conclusion, the benefits of whole grains are numerous and well-documented. From promoting digestive health to reducing our risk of chronic diseases, incorporating whole grains into our diet can have a significant impact on our overall health and well-being. By choosing whole grain products and incorporating them into our meals and snacks, we can enjoy their many health benefits while also enjoying delicious and nutritious food.

Chapter 39: The Benefits of Healthy Fats

Healthy fats are a crucial part of a well-balanced diet. They play a crucial role in many physiological processes in the body, from building cell membranes to hormone production. While it might seem counterintuitive, consuming healthy fats in moderation can actually help you maintain a healthy weight and reduce your risk of chronic diseases like heart disease, diabetes, and cancer.

One of the primary benefits of healthy fats is their ability to help you feel fuller for longer periods of time. Unlike carbohydrates, which can cause blood sugar levels to spike and then crash, fats take longer to digest and help regulate appetite. This means that consuming healthy fats can help you maintain a healthier weight by reducing the likelihood of overeating or snacking between meals.

In addition to helping regulate appetite, healthy fats also play a crucial role in brain function. The brain is made up of approximately 60% fat, and consuming healthy fats can help support healthy brain function and prevent cognitive decline. Omega-3 fatty acids, in particular, are important for brain health, and studies have shown that increasing omega-3 intake can improve memory, concentration, and overall cognitive function.

Healthy fats are also important for heart health. While consuming too much saturated fat can increase your risk of heart disease, consuming healthy fats like monounsaturated and polyunsaturated fats can actually help reduce your risk. These fats can help lower LDL (bad) cholesterol levels and reduce inflammation, both of which are major contributors to heart disease.

Another important benefit of healthy fats is their ability to support healthy skin, hair, and nails. Fats help keep skin hydrated, which can prevent dryness and wrinkles. They also help support hair and nail growth and strength, which can be particularly important as we age.

There are many sources of healthy fats, including avocados, nuts, seeds, fatty fish, and olive oil. It's important to choose healthy fats in moderation and to avoid processed or fried foods that are high in unhealthy fats. Incorporating healthy fats into your diet can have a wide range of health benefits, from supporting heart and brain health to improving skin and hair health.

Chapter 40: The Benefits of Herbs and Spices

Herbs and spices have been used in cooking and traditional medicine for thousands of years, and for good reason. These plant-based ingredients offer numerous health benefits, as well as adding delicious flavors and aromas to food. In this chapter, we'll explore some of the many benefits of herbs and spices.

Anti-inflammatory properties

Many herbs and spices have anti-inflammatory properties, which can help reduce inflammation in the body. Chronic inflammation has been linked to a range of health problems, including heart disease, cancer, and diabetes. Some examples of anti-inflammatory herbs and spices include turmeric, ginger, garlic, and cinnamon.

Antioxidant effects

Herbs and spices are rich in antioxidants, which help protect the body from damage caused by free radicals. Free radicals are unstable molecules that can damage cells and contribute to aging and disease. Antioxidants neutralize these molecules and prevent or repair damage to cells. Examples of antioxidant-rich herbs and spices include oregano, thyme, basil, and rosemary.

Digestive health

Many herbs and spices can help promote healthy digestion. For example, ginger and peppermint have been shown to help relieve nausea and other digestive symptoms. Fennel and coriander can also help ease digestive discomfort and improve digestion.

Blood sugar control

Some herbs and spices have been shown to help regulate blood sugar levels, which can be especially beneficial for people with diabetes or at risk of developing it. Cinnamon, for example, has been shown to improve insulin sensitivity and lower blood sugar levels.

Immune system support

Several herbs and spices have immune-boosting properties, which can help the body fight off infections and illnesses. Garlic, for example, has antimicrobial properties and may help prevent colds and flu. Echinacea is another herb that is often used to support the immune system and prevent or treat colds.

Brain health

Some herbs and spices may have cognitive benefits, such as improving memory and concentration. Rosemary, for example, has been shown to improve memory and mental performance in some studies. Turmeric has also been studied for its potential to improve cognitive function and prevent age-related decline.

Incorporating herbs and spices into your diet is easy and delicious. You can use them to add flavor to soups, stews, marinades, and dressings. You can also experiment with different blends of herbs and spices to create your own unique flavors. Whether you're looking to improve your health or simply add some variety to your meals, herbs and spices are a great way to do it.

Chapter 41: Cooking Methods for Healthy Eating

Eating healthy is not just about the foods you choose, but also how you prepare them. Cooking methods can greatly impact the nutritional value of your meals, and choosing the right techniques can help you maximize the health benefits of the ingredients you use. In this chapter, we will explore some cooking methods that are ideal for healthy eating.

Grilling

Grilling is a popular cooking method that can be very healthy if done correctly. When you grill, you cook your food over an open flame or high heat, which can help to reduce the fat content of the food by allowing excess fat to drip away. Grilling is also a great way to add flavor to your food without the use of additional fats or oils.

To make the most of grilling, choose lean cuts of meat and vegetables. Marinate your meat or veggies beforehand to add flavor and moisture, and avoid charring your food, which can create potentially harmful compounds. Instead, aim to cook your food until it is lightly charred and cooked to your desired level of doneness.

Steaming

Steaming is a gentle cooking method that helps to retain the nutrients in your food while also reducing the amount of fat needed for cooking. Steaming involves cooking food over boiling water, either in a steamer basket or in a covered pot with a small amount of water.

To steam food, simply place it in the steamer basket or pot, and cook until tender. Steaming is a great way to cook vegetables, as it helps to preserve their color, flavor, and nutritional content. You can also steam fish, poultry, and other meats for a healthy and delicious meal.

Baking

Baking is a healthy cooking method that can be used to cook a wide variety of foods. When you bake, you cook your food in the oven, either on a baking sheet or in a covered dish. Baking is a great way to cook foods like chicken, fish, and vegetables, as it helps to retain their nutrients and flavor.

To bake healthy meals, choose lean cuts of meat and use herbs and spices to add flavor instead of using high-fat sauces or gravies. You can also bake healthy desserts, like fruit crisps or baked apples, using natural sweeteners like honey or maple syrup.

Stir-frying

Stir-frying is a quick and easy cooking method that can be used to cook a variety of healthy meals. When you stir-fry, you cook your food in a small amount of oil over high heat, stirring constantly to prevent burning.

To stir-fry healthy meals, use a non-stick pan or wok and choose lean cuts of meat or tofu. Add plenty of vegetables, like broccoli, peppers, and mushrooms, for added nutrients and flavor. Use flavorful sauces like soy sauce, garlic, and ginger, instead of high-fat sauces, to add flavor to your stir-fry.

Poaching

Poaching is a healthy cooking method that involves cooking food in liquid, like water or broth, at a low temperature. Poaching is a great way to cook delicate foods like fish, chicken, and eggs, as it helps to retain their moisture and flavor.

To poach healthy meals, use low-sodium broth or water, and add flavorful herbs and spices, like bay leaves or thyme, to the cooking liquid. Poach lean cuts of meat or fish until they are tender and fully cooked.

In conclusion, choosing healthy cooking methods can help you to create delicious, nutritious meals that support your overall health and well-being. Experiment with these techniques and find the ones that work best for you and your family.

Chapter 42: Healthy Eating on a Budget

Eating healthy can be a challenge, especially when you're on a tight budget. However, it's important to remember that healthy eating doesn't always mean expensive food. By making a few changes to your grocery shopping and meal planning habits, you can eat healthy and stay within your budget.

Plan Your Meals

One of the best ways to save money and eat healthy is by planning your meals. Start by creating a weekly meal plan that includes all of your breakfasts, lunches, dinners, and snacks for the week. This will help you stay on track and avoid impulse purchases when you go grocery shopping.

Buy in Bulk

Buying in bulk can be a great way to save money on healthy foods. Look for bulk bins at your grocery store or buy larger packages of items like rice, beans, and nuts. These foods are typically less expensive in bulk and can be stored in airtight containers for extended periods.

Shop Seasonal

Seasonal produce is not only fresher and more flavorful, but it's also typically less expensive. Check your local farmer's market or grocery store for seasonal fruits and vegetables. You can also freeze or can these foods to enjoy them year-round.

Stick to the Basics

You don't have to buy expensive superfoods or specialty products to eat healthy. Stick to the basics like fruits, vegetables, whole grains, and lean protein sources like chicken, turkey, and beans. These foods are not only affordable but also packed with essential nutrients.

Cook at Home

Eating out can quickly add up and be a drain on your budget. Cooking at home not only saves money but also allows you to control the ingredients and portion sizes in your meals. Invest in some basic kitchen equipment like a good knife and cutting board, and start experimenting with healthy recipes.

Choose Affordable Protein Sources

Protein is an essential part of a healthy diet, but it can also be expensive. Look for affordable protein sources like eggs, canned tuna, tofu, and lentils. These foods are not only affordable but also versatile and can be used in a variety of dishes.

In conclusion, eating healthy on a budget is possible with a little planning and smart shopping. By focusing on whole, nutrient-dense foods and preparing meals at home, you can improve your health and save money at the same time. Remember to prioritize the basics, buy in bulk, shop seasonally, and choose affordable protein sources to make the most of your grocery budget.

Chapter 43: Healthy Eating for Busy People

Eating healthy is important for everyone, but it can be particularly challenging for busy individuals who are constantly on the go. Whether you are a busy parent, a student with a full schedule, or a professional with a demanding job, finding the time to plan and prepare healthy meals can be a struggle. However, with a few simple strategies and some smart choices, it is possible to maintain a healthy diet even when you are short on time.

Plan Ahead

One of the most effective ways to ensure that you are eating healthy is to plan your meals in advance. Take a few minutes at the beginning of each week to plan out your meals for the upcoming days. This will help you stay organized and ensure that you have healthy food options available when you need them.

Pack Your Lunch

If you are someone who eats lunch on the go, packing your lunch is a great way to make sure that you are eating healthy. Bring along some fresh fruits and vegetables, lean proteins like grilled chicken or fish, and whole-grain bread or pasta. Not only will this help you eat healthier, but it can also save you money and time.

Stock Up on Healthy Snacks

When you are busy, it can be tempting to grab unhealthy snacks on the go. However, by keeping healthy snacks on hand, you can avoid the temptation of junk food. Stock up on items like fresh fruit, nuts, seeds, and whole-grain crackers. These snacks are portable and easy to grab when you are on the go.

Use Your Slow Cooker

If you don't have a lot of time to spend in the kitchen, a slow cooker can be your best friend. Simply toss in some healthy ingredients like lean meats, vegetables, and whole grains, and let the slow cooker do the work for you. When you get home at the end of the day, you will have a healthy, home-cooked meal waiting for you.

Make Healthy Choices When Eating Out

When you are busy, it can be tempting to grab food on the go. However, many fast food options are high in calories, fat, and sodium. If you do need to eat out, look for healthier options like salads, grilled chicken, or vegetable-based dishes. You can also check the nutrition information online before you go, so you know what you are getting into.

Keep It Simple

When it comes to healthy eating, it doesn't have to be complicated. Focus on simple, whole foods like fresh fruits and vegetables, lean proteins, and whole grains. By keeping your meals simple, you can save time and ensure that you are getting the nutrients your body needs.

In conclusion, eating healthy can be a challenge for busy people, but it is possible with some planning and smart choices. By packing your lunch, stocking up on healthy snacks, using your slow cooker, making healthy choices when eating out, and keeping your meals simple, you can maintain a healthy diet even when you are short on time.

Chapter 44: Healthy Eating for Kids

As a parent or caregiver, you play an essential role in shaping your child's eating habits. Teaching children the importance of healthy eating at a young age can have a significant impact on their overall health and well-being. In this chapter, we'll explore some tips and tricks for promoting healthy eating for kids.

Lead by example

Children learn by watching their parents and caregivers. So, it's essential to model healthy eating habits yourself. If your child sees you eating fruits, vegetables, and whole grains, they are more likely to follow suit. Make sure to eat together as a family and avoid skipping meals, especially breakfast, which is the most important meal of the day.

Get creative with healthy foods

Kids can be picky eaters, but there are many ways to make healthy foods more appealing to them. For example, you can cut fruits and vegetables into fun shapes or use dips like hummus or guacamole. You can also involve your child in meal preparation, such as letting them pick out fruits and vegetables at the grocery store or helping them make a healthy snack.

Limit processed and sugary foods

Processed and sugary foods can be high in calories and low in nutrients, leading to weight gain and other health problems. Try to limit your child's intake of these foods and instead focus on whole, nutrient-dense foods like fruits, vegetables, whole grains, and lean proteins.

Make sure they drink enough water

Water is essential for staying hydrated and supporting overall health. Encourage your child to drink water throughout the day and limit their intake of sugary drinks like soda and juice.

Teach moderation

It's okay to indulge in treats once in a while, but it's important to teach your child about moderation. Explain that treats should be enjoyed in moderation and that a balanced diet is essential for good health.

In summary, promoting healthy eating for kids involves modeling healthy habits, getting creative with healthy foods, limiting processed and sugary foods, making sure they drink enough water, and teaching moderation. By following these tips, you can help your child develop healthy eating habits that will benefit them throughout their life.

Chapter 45: Healthy Eating for Pregnant Women

Pregnancy is a time of major changes in a woman's body and it is important to maintain a healthy diet to support both the mother and the developing fetus. Eating well during pregnancy can help ensure that the baby grows and develops properly, and can also reduce the risk of complications for the mother.

Here are some guidelines to follow for healthy eating during pregnancy:

Eat a balanced diet

A balanced diet should include a variety of foods from all food groups, including fruits and vegetables, whole grains, lean proteins, and healthy fats. Aim to eat a rainbow of colors to ensure that you are getting a variety of vitamins and minerals.

Get enough protein

Protein is essential for building and repairing tissues, and is especially important during pregnancy when the body is building the baby's organs and tissues. Good sources of protein include lean meats, poultry, fish, beans, lentils, nuts, and seeds.

Choose healthy fats

Healthy fats are important for the development of the baby's brain and nervous system. Good sources of healthy fats include fatty fish, nuts, seeds, avocado, and olive oil.

Avoid certain foods

Some foods should be avoided during pregnancy due to the risk of foodborne illness or other complications. These include raw or undercooked meat, poultry, and fish, unpasteurized dairy products, raw sprouts, and some types of fish that are high in mercury.

Stay hydrated

Drinking enough water is important during pregnancy to support the increased blood volume and amniotic fluid.

Aim for at least 8-10 cups of water per day, and drink more if you are exercising or in hot weather.

Take prenatal vitamins

Prenatal vitamins are important for ensuring that you are getting enough of the vitamins and minerals needed for a healthy pregnancy. Be sure to talk to your doctor about which prenatal vitamins are best for you.

Listen to your body

Pregnancy can cause changes in appetite and cravings, and it's important to listen to your body's signals. Eat when you are hungry and stop when you are full. Don't worry too much about weight gain, as it is normal and healthy to gain weight during pregnancy.

In conclusion, a healthy diet is essential for a healthy pregnancy. By following these guidelines and listening to your body's needs, you can help ensure a healthy pregnancy and a healthy baby. Be sure to talk to your doctor or a registered dietitian if you have any concerns or questions about your diet during pregnancy.

Chapter 46: Healthy Eating for Athletes

Athletes require a balanced and healthy diet to maintain their energy levels and enhance their physical performance. The body needs the right balance of nutrients and calories to perform at its best. Here are some key principles of healthy eating for athletes:

Eat a Balanced Diet

A balanced diet for athletes should include carbohydrates, proteins, and fats. Carbohydrates are the body's primary source of energy, while protein helps to build and repair muscle tissue. Fats are also essential for energy, hormone production, and maintaining cell health. Aim to consume a variety of foods from all food groups to ensure a balanced diet.

Carbohydrates are Key

Carbohydrates are the primary fuel source for athletes, especially those engaged in endurance activities. The body converts carbohydrates into glycogen, which is stored in the muscles and liver for energy during physical activity. Carbohydrates can be found in foods such as whole grains, fruits, vegetables, and legumes. Aim to consume a variety of carbohydrate-rich foods before, during, and after exercise to maintain energy levels.

Protein for Muscle Repair

Protein is essential for building and repairing muscle tissue, making it crucial for athletes. Protein can be found in foods such as meat, fish, eggs, dairy, and plant-based sources such as beans and lentils. Aim to consume protein-rich foods throughout the day to support muscle growth and repair.

Don't Forget the Fat

Fats are an essential part of a healthy diet and are essential for energy production and hormone regulation. Choose healthy sources of fats such as nuts, seeds, avocado, and fatty fish. Limit saturated and trans fats found in processed and fried foods.

Stay Hydrated

Athletes need to stay hydrated to maintain their performance levels. Aim to drink water before, during, and after exercise to replenish lost fluids. Sports drinks can also be useful for prolonged endurance activities lasting more than an hour.

Timing is Everything

When and how much you eat is just as important as what you eat. Timing your meals and snacks around your training schedule can help maintain energy levels and aid in muscle recovery. Aim to eat a meal containing carbohydrates and protein two to three hours before exercise and a small snack containing carbohydrates 30 minutes to an hour before exercise. After exercise, aim to consume a meal containing carbohydrates and protein within 30 minutes to aid in muscle recovery.

Supplements

While a balanced diet should provide all the necessary nutrients for athletes, some may benefit from supplements such as vitamins, minerals, and protein powders. Consult with a sports dietitian to determine if supplements are necessary and to develop a safe and effective supplement plan.

In summary, a healthy diet for athletes should include a variety of foods from all food groups, with an emphasis on carbohydrates, protein, and healthy fats. Timing meals and snacks around training sessions is crucial for maintaining energy levels and aiding in muscle recovery. Adequate hydration is also essential for optimal performance. Finally, consult with a sports dietitian to develop a personalized nutrition plan that meets your individual needs.

Chapter 47: Healthy Eating for Vegetarians and Vegans

Eating a healthy diet is essential for overall wellbeing, and for those following a vegetarian or vegan lifestyle, it can sometimes feel daunting to ensure that all essential nutrients are included in their diets. However, with the right planning and knowledge, it is entirely possible to maintain a balanced and healthy diet while following a plant-based lifestyle. In this chapter, we will explore the essential nutrients that vegetarians and vegans should be aware of, as well as practical tips for incorporating them into their diets.

Protein

Protein is essential for maintaining and building muscle, and it is often a concern for those following a vegetarian or vegan diet. However, there are plenty of plant-based sources of protein, including beans, lentils, chickpeas, tofu, tempeh, seitan, nuts, and seeds. It is essential to include a variety of protein sources in your diet to ensure that you are getting all of the essential amino acids.

Iron

Iron is vital for producing red blood cells and transporting oxygen throughout the body. While red meat is an excellent source of iron, vegetarians and vegans can obtain it from plant-based sources such as leafy greens, beans, lentils, tofu, tempeh, fortified cereals, and dried fruit. It is important to note that iron from plant-based sources is not as easily absorbed by the body as iron from animal sources, so it is important to consume these foods with vitamin C-rich foods, such as citrus fruits or tomatoes, to increase absorption.

Calcium

Calcium is essential for building and maintaining strong bones and teeth. While dairy products are a good source of calcium, vegetarians and vegans can obtain it from plant-based sources such as leafy greens, fortified plant milk, tofu, and almonds. It is important to consume enough calcium daily to maintain bone health.

Vitamin B12

Vitamin B12 is necessary for proper nerve function and the production of red blood cells. It is only found naturally in animal products, so vegetarians and vegans must obtain it from fortified foods, such as plant milk, breakfast cereals, and nutritional yeast, or through supplements.

Omega-3 Fatty Acids

Omega-3 fatty acids are essential for brain function and heart health. While fatty fish is a good source of omega-3s, vegetarians and vegans can obtain them from plant-based sources such as flaxseeds, chia seeds, walnuts, and hemp seeds.

Practical Tips for Incorporating These Nutrients into Your Diet

One of the most important things you can do to ensure that you are getting all of the necessary nutrients in your diet is to eat a varied diet that includes a wide range of whole, plant-based foods. Here are some practical tips for incorporating these essential nutrients into your diet:

Include a source of protein at every meal and snack, such as beans, tofu, or nuts.

Choose leafy greens as a source of calcium, such as kale, bok choy, or collard greens.

Fortify your plant milk with calcium and vitamin D.

Include a source of vitamin C with iron-rich foods, such as a glass of orange juice with your breakfast cereal.

Consider taking a vitamin B12 supplement or eating fortified foods.

Add ground flaxseeds to your morning smoothie or sprinkle them on your oatmeal for a boost of omega-3s.

In conclusion, a healthy vegetarian or vegan diet can provide all of the necessary nutrients for optimal health. By including a variety of plant-based foods in your diet and being mindful of essential nutrients such as protein, iron, calcium, vitamin B12, and omega-3 fatty acids, you can enjoy a nutritious and satisfying diet while reaping the many benefits of a plant-based lifestyle.

Chapter 48: Healthy Eating When Dining Out

Eating out is a common part of modern life, but it can pose challenges to maintaining a healthy diet. Dining out often means indulging in high-calorie dishes that are loaded with unhealthy fats, sugars, and sodium. However, it is possible to enjoy a meal out while still sticking to a healthy eating plan. Here are some tips for making smart choices when dining out:

Research menus ahead of time

Many restaurants now publish their menus online, which means you can check out the options before you arrive. Look for dishes that are lower in calories and fat, such as grilled chicken, fish, or vegetables. Avoid anything that is fried or comes with heavy sauces or cheese.

Watch portion sizes

Restaurant portions tend to be much larger than what you would normally eat at home. To avoid overeating, ask for a to-go box at the beginning of the meal and immediately put half of your meal in the box to take home. This way, you can enjoy your meal without feeling guilty or overeating.

Choose healthier sides

Many restaurants offer healthier side dishes, such as salads or grilled vegetables, instead of fries or mashed potatoes. If you do want a starchy side dish, choose brown rice or sweet potatoes instead of white rice or regular potatoes.

Be mindful of drinks

Sugary drinks like soda, sweet tea, or lemonade can quickly add up in calories and sugar. Opt for water or unsweetened tea instead. If you must have a drink with flavor, choose a low-calorie option like a flavored sparkling water.

Avoid bread baskets

Many restaurants serve bread or rolls before the meal, but these are often high in calories and refined carbohydrates. Avoid the bread basket altogether, or limit yourself to one small piece.

Customize your order

Don't be afraid to ask the server to make adjustments to your meal. Ask for dressing on the side, request grilled instead of fried, or substitute a side for a healthier option. Many restaurants are happy to accommodate special requests.

Don't skip meals

Many people make the mistake of skipping meals in anticipation of a big restaurant meal. However, this can lead to overeating and poor choices. Instead, eat a healthy snack or meal before you go out to eat, so you are not ravenous when you arrive.

Focus on enjoying the experience

Remember that dining out is not just about the food; it's also about the experience. Enjoy the company of your friends or family, take your time, and savor your meal. By focusing on the social aspect of dining out, you are less likely to overindulge or make poor choices.

By following these tips, you can enjoy a meal out while still maintaining a healthy diet. With a little bit of planning and mindfulness, you can make healthy choices even when dining out.

Chapter 49: Reading Food Labels

When it comes to healthy eating, understanding how to read food labels is an essential skill. Food labels contain important information about the nutritional content of the food you are buying, which can help you make informed decisions about what you eat. Here are some key things to look for when reading food labels.

Serving size: The first thing to look for on a food label is the serving size. This is the amount of the food that the label is referring to. All of the other nutritional information on the label is based on this serving size. Make sure to pay attention to the serving size so that you can accurately calculate the nutritional content of the food you are eating.

Calories: Calories are a measure of the amount of energy in a food. It is important to pay attention to the number of calories in a serving, especially if you are trying to manage your weight. If you are trying to lose weight, you may want to choose foods that are lower in calories.

Fat: Fat is an important part of a healthy diet, but some types of fat are better for you than others. Look for foods that are low in saturated and trans fats and high in unsaturated fats, such as omega-3 fatty acids. Saturated and trans fats can increase your risk of heart disease, while unsaturated fats can help improve your heart health.

Sodium: Sodium is a mineral that is found in many foods. While sodium is important for your body, too much sodium can increase your blood pressure and your risk of heart disease. Look for foods that are low in sodium, especially if you are trying to manage your blood pressure.

Carbohydrates: Carbohydrates are a major source of energy for your body. Look for foods that are high in fiber and low in added sugars. Fiber can help keep you feeling full and can help lower your risk of heart disease and diabetes, while added sugars can contribute to weight gain and other health problems.

Protein: Protein is important for building and repairing your muscles and tissues. Look for foods that are high in protein, especially if you are trying to build muscle or recover from an injury. However, it is important to remember that not all sources of protein are created equal. Choose lean sources of protein, such as chicken, fish, and beans, over high-fat sources of protein, such as bacon and sausage.

In addition to these key components, food labels may also contain information about vitamins, minerals, and other nutrients. By understanding how to read food labels, you can make informed decisions about the foods you eat and improve your overall health and well-being.

Chapter 50: The Dangers of Processed Foods

In today's fast-paced world, it's no surprise that many people rely on processed foods for quick and convenient meals. However, while these foods may be convenient, they come with a host of dangers that can impact your health in both the short and long term. In this chapter, we will explore the dangers of processed foods and why you should avoid them as much as possible.

Processed foods are defined as foods that have been altered from their natural state through various methods, such as cooking, preserving, or adding chemicals and artificial ingredients. These foods are often high in calories, unhealthy fats, sugar, and salt, and low in essential nutrients like vitamins, minerals, and fiber.

One of the most significant dangers of processed foods is their negative impact on our health. Consuming too many processed foods can lead to weight gain, obesity, and a host of related health issues like diabetes, high blood pressure, and heart disease. Processed foods are often high in sugar, which can lead to insulin resistance, a condition where the body's cells don't respond to insulin properly, leading to high blood sugar levels.

Processed foods are also often high in unhealthy fats like trans fats and saturated fats, which can increase your risk of heart disease and other health issues. Additionally, many processed foods contain high levels of sodium, which can contribute to high blood pressure, heart disease, and stroke.

Another danger of processed foods is their impact on our gut health. Many processed foods contain preservatives and other chemicals that can disrupt the balance of bacteria in our gut, leading to digestive issues like bloating, gas, and constipation. A healthy gut is essential for overall health, so it's crucial to avoid foods that can disrupt its delicate balance.

Processed foods can also be addictive, leading to cravings and overconsumption. Many processed foods are designed to be hyper-palatable, meaning they are engineered to be so delicious that we can't resist them. This can lead to overeating and weight gain, which can further exacerbate the health issues associated with processed foods.

In conclusion, while processed foods may be convenient and tasty, they come with a host of dangers that can impact our health in both the short and long term. To maintain optimal health, it's essential to limit your consumption of processed foods and opt for whole, natural foods as much as possible. By making healthy choices, you can support your overall well-being and live a vibrant, healthy life.

Chapter 51: The Dangers of Added Sugars

When we think about unhealthy foods, we often think of items like fried foods, fast food, and processed snacks. However, one of the biggest culprits of poor health is something that many of us consume on a daily basis: added sugars.

Added sugars are any sugars that are added to food or drink during processing, preparation, or at the table. This includes common sweeteners like table sugar, corn syrup, honey, and maple syrup. Unfortunately, added sugars are found in a wide variety of products, from sodas and candy to bread and salad dressings.

One of the biggest dangers of added sugars is their impact on our weight. Consuming too many added sugars can lead to weight gain and obesity, which in turn increases the risk of many health problems, including type 2 diabetes, heart disease, and certain cancers. Added sugars also provide empty calories, which means they offer little to no nutritional value but still contribute to overall calorie intake.

Another danger of added sugars is their impact on our energy levels. While sugary snacks may give us a quick burst of energy, this is often followed by a crash. Consuming too much sugar can also disrupt our body's natural energy systems, leading to fatigue and a lack of motivation.

In addition to these physical effects, added sugars can also have an impact on our mental health. Studies have shown that a diet high in added sugars may contribute to anxiety, depression, and even cognitive decline. This may be due to the way that sugar affects our brain chemistry and the inflammation it can cause throughout the body.

So, what can we do to reduce our intake of added sugars? The easiest way is to read labels and be mindful of the foods we consume. Look for products that are low in added sugars, and try to choose whole foods instead of processed snacks. It's also important to be aware of the many hidden sources of added sugars, such as ketchup, BBQ sauce, and fruit juice.

Ultimately, reducing our intake of added sugars is an important step towards a healthier lifestyle. By making small changes to our diet and being mindful of the foods we consume, we can improve our overall health and reduce the risk of many chronic diseases.

Chapter 52: The Dangers of Artificial Sweeteners

Artificial sweeteners have become increasingly popular in recent years, as people look for ways to reduce their sugar intake without sacrificing sweetness in their diet. However, despite their popularity, there are a number of potential dangers associated with these sweeteners that are important to consider.

One of the main concerns with artificial sweeteners is their impact on weight and metabolism. While these sweeteners may not contain calories, studies have shown that they can still have an effect on the body's insulin response and metabolism. In fact, some research has suggested that regular consumption of artificial sweeteners may actually lead to weight gain and an increased risk of metabolic syndrome.

Another danger of artificial sweeteners is their impact on gut health. Studies have shown that these sweeteners can alter the balance of bacteria in the gut, leading to negative effects on digestion and overall health. Some studies have even suggested that regular consumption of artificial sweeteners may increase the risk of inflammatory bowel disease.

In addition to these health concerns, there are also questions surrounding the safety of some artificial sweeteners. For example, aspartame has been the subject of controversy for many years, with some studies suggesting that it may be linked to an increased risk of cancer. While these claims have not been definitively proven, they have led some experts to question the safety of this and other artificial sweeteners.

Despite these dangers, many people continue to use artificial sweeteners as a way to reduce their sugar intake. While it's true that reducing sugar consumption is important for overall health, there are other ways to do so without relying on artificial sweeteners. For example, incorporating more whole foods into your diet, such as fruits and vegetables, can help to naturally reduce your sugar intake while providing a wide range of other health benefits.

Ultimately, while artificial sweeteners may seem like an appealing option for those looking to reduce their sugar intake, the potential dangers associated with these sweeteners should not be ignored. By taking a more natural approach to reducing sugar intake and focusing on whole foods, you can enjoy a healthy diet without putting your health at risk.

Chapter 53: The Dangers of Trans Fats

Trans fats, also known as partially hydrogenated oils, are a type of unsaturated fat that have been chemically altered to increase their shelf life and stability. They are commonly found in processed foods such as fried foods, baked goods, snack foods, and margarine. While trans fats were once considered a healthier alternative to saturated fats, research has now shown that they are actually incredibly harmful to our health.

One of the biggest dangers of trans fats is their effect on our cardiovascular health. Studies have found that consuming trans fats can raise levels of LDL (or "bad") cholesterol while lowering levels of HDL (or "good") cholesterol, increasing the risk of heart disease, stroke, and other cardiovascular problems. In fact, the American Heart Association recommends that people consume as little trans fat as possible, with an ideal intake of zero grams per day.

In addition to their impact on heart health, trans fats have also been linked to other negative health outcomes. Studies have found that consuming trans fats can increase inflammation throughout the body, leading to a range of health problems including insulin resistance, type 2 diabetes, and even certain types of cancer. Trans fats have also been found to negatively impact brain health, with some studies linking them to a higher risk of Alzheimer's disease and other cognitive disorders.

Perhaps one of the most concerning aspects of trans fats is that they are often hidden in processed foods, making it difficult for consumers to know exactly how much they are consuming. In fact, until recently, trans fats were not even required to be listed on food labels. While this has changed in many countries, it is still important for consumers to carefully read labels and look for products that are labeled as "trans fat-free" or "no trans fats."

Fortunately, there are many healthier alternatives to trans fats that can be used in cooking and baking. These include plant-based oils such as olive, canola, and avocado oil, as well as natural sources of saturated fat like coconut oil and grass-fed butter. By making a conscious effort to avoid trans fats and opt for healthier alternatives, we can protect our cardiovascular health and overall wellbeing.

Chapter 54: The Dangers of Excessive Salt Intake

Salt is an essential ingredient in cooking, and it is commonly used to enhance the flavor of food. However, consuming too much salt can have serious health consequences. The average American consumes approximately 3,400 mg of sodium per day, which is more than double the recommended daily intake of 1,500-2,300 mg of sodium.

Excessive salt intake can lead to high blood pressure, which is a major risk factor for heart disease, stroke, and kidney disease. When you consume too much salt, your body retains water to dilute the excess sodium in your blood. This can lead to an increase in blood volume, which puts additional strain on your heart and blood vessels. Over time, this can lead to damage to your blood vessels, which can cause them to become less flexible and more prone to blockages.

In addition to its effects on the cardiovascular system, excessive salt intake can also have negative impacts on other areas of your health. For example, it can contribute to the development of osteoporosis by leaching calcium from your bones. It can also increase the risk of stomach cancer, as well as other digestive problems like ulcers and acid reflux.

One of the challenges of reducing salt intake is that salt is often hidden in processed and packaged foods. Many pre-packaged meals, snacks, and even drinks contain high levels of sodium, making it difficult to know how much you are consuming. Additionally, some people are more sensitive to the effects of salt than others, meaning that even small amounts can have a significant impact on their health.

There are several steps you can take to reduce your salt intake and protect your health. First, try to eat more fresh fruits and vegetables, which are naturally low in sodium. When cooking, use herbs and spices to add flavor instead of relying on salt. If you do use salt, opt for a high-quality sea salt or kosher salt, which have a more complex flavor than table salt and can be used in smaller amounts. When shopping for packaged foods, read labels carefully and look for products that are low in sodium.

In conclusion, excessive salt intake can have serious health consequences, including high blood pressure, heart disease, stroke, kidney disease, osteoporosis, and digestive problems. By being mindful of your salt intake and taking steps to reduce it, you can protect your health and enjoy the benefits of a diet that is rich in fresh, whole foods.

Chapter 55: Conclusion and Action Steps for a Healthier You

Congratulations! By reading this book, you have taken an important step towards a healthier lifestyle. Eating healthy is not just about losing weight, but it is also about feeling better, having more energy, and reducing the risk of chronic diseases. Now that you have learned about the benefits of healthy eating, it is time to take action.

Here are some action steps that you can take to improve your eating habits:

Plan Your Meals

Planning your meals is a great way to ensure that you eat healthy foods. Make a list of healthy foods that you enjoy and plan your meals for the week. This will save you time and money, and it will help you avoid unhealthy food choices when you are hungry and in a rush.

Eat More Fruits and Vegetables

Fruits and vegetables are packed with vitamins, minerals, and fiber. They are low in calories and can help you feel full for longer periods of time. Try to include a variety of fruits and vegetables in your meals and snacks. Aim for at least five servings a day.

Choose Whole Grains

Whole grains are rich in fiber and other nutrients that are important for good health. Choose whole grain bread, rice, pasta, and cereals instead of refined grains. Look for products that are labeled as 100% whole grain or whole wheat.

Limit Processed Foods

Processed foods are often high in sugar, salt, and unhealthy fats. They can contribute to weight gain and increase the risk of chronic diseases. Try to limit your intake of processed foods and opt for fresh, whole foods instead.

Drink Plenty of Water

Water is essential for good health. It helps to keep your body hydrated and can aid in weight loss. Aim for at least eight glasses of water a day, and avoid sugary drinks.

Practice Mindful Eating

Mindful eating involves paying attention to your food and the experience of eating. It can help you develop a healthier relationship with food and avoid overeating. Take time to savor your food and listen to your body's hunger and fullness signals.

Stay Active

Physical activity is essential for good health. It can help you maintain a healthy weight, reduce the risk of chronic diseases, and improve your mood. Aim for at least 30 minutes of moderate-intensity exercise most days of the week.

In conclusion, eating healthy is one of the best things you can do for your health. By making simple changes to your eating habits, you can improve your overall well-being and reduce the risk of chronic diseases. Remember to plan your meals, eat more fruits and vegetables, choose whole grains, limit processed foods, drink plenty of water, practice mindful eating, and stay active. With these action steps, you can achieve a healthier you!